DERMATOLOGY - LABORATORY AND CLINICAL RESEARCH

PEMPHIGUS VULGARIS

SCIENTIFIC BASIS, CLINICAL PRESENTATIONS, DIAGNOSTIC METHODOLOGY AND MANAGEMENT STRATEGIES

DERMATOLOGY - LABORATORY AND CLINICAL RESEARCH

Additional books in this series can be found on Nova's website under the Series tab.

Additional e-books in this series can be found on Nova's website under the e-book tab.

DERMATOLOGY - LABORATORY AND CLINICAL RESEARCH

PEMPHIGUS VULGARIS

SCIENTIFIC BASIS, CLINICAL PRESENTATIONS, DIAGNOSTIC METHODOLOGY AND MANAGEMENT STRATEGIES

LAWRENCE S. CHAN

New York

NOTICE TO THE READER

Library of Congress Cataloging-in-Publication Data

ISBN: 978-1-63484-307-2

Library of Congress Control Number: 2015957367

Published by Nova Science Publishers, Inc. † New York

Contents

Preface

This book gathers all up-to-date information regarding the historical perspectives, clinical manifestations, pathomechanism, diagnostic methodology, and therapeutic strategies for a life-threatening, blistering skin disease called *pemphigus vulgaris*. The medical community has come a long way in discovering its disease mechanism down to the molecular level and found excellent treatment options for patients suffering from this horrific disease. Compared to the pre-corticosteroid era when the mortality rate was greater than 90% to present day mortality, which is extremely rare, the medical community have indeed made great medical progress toward curing this disease. The scientific and clinical advancements notwithstanding, patients affected by this disease still face a mortality rate two to three times higher than the general population, indicating that the research of this disease has not yet been completed. While this book is focused on *pemphigus vulgaris*, it also includes four clinical variants of *pemphigus vulgaris*: drug-induced pemphigus, paraneoplastic pemphigus, pemphigus vegetans, and IgA pemphigus. Accompanied with extensive reviews of scientific literature are clinical photos illustrating the various clinical presentations of the disease, as well as histological and immunohistological patterns of this disease that would serve as outstanding references for practical usage in emergency rooms, hospitals, and outpatient clinics. This book is intended for: medical students whom require comprehensive knowledge of a well-classified organ-specific autoimmune disease; dermatology residents solidifying their ability to diagnose and treat this group of patients; practicing physicians whom need to update their skills in managing patients suffering from this disease; emergency physicians in order to properly triage their patients; scientists completing their understanding of the disease pathophysiology; and pharmaceutical industries searching for even better treatment options for these patients.

Lawrence S. Chan
University of Illinois College of Medicine,
Chicago, IL
larrycha@uic.edu

Acknowledgments

This work is in part supported by Dr. Orville J. Stone Professorship. The author wishes to thank Dr. Iris K. Aronson for many of her collection of clinical photos.

List of Abbreviations

PV	pemphigus vulgaris
PF	pemphigus foliaceus
BP	bullous pemphigoid
DIF	direct immunofluorescence microscopy
IgG	immunoglobulin G
IIF	indirect immunofluorescence Microscopy
IV	intravenous
IVIg	intravenous immunoglobulin
PNP	paraneoplastic pemphigus
Dsg	desmoglein
AZA	azathioprine
MMF	mycophenolate mofetil
CYC	cyclophosphamide
MTX	methotrexate
CSP	cyclosporine
RTX	rituximab
IFX	infliximab
HLA	human leukocyte antigen
APC	antigen presenting cell
TCR	T cell receptor
MAPK	mitogen-activated protein kinase
EGFR	epidermal growth factor receptor
H-CDR3	heavy chain complementarity-determining region 3
OCT	optimal cutting temperature
SNP	single-nucleotide polymorphisms

TPMT	thiopurine S-methyltransferase
ITPA	inosine triphosphate pyrophosphohydrolase

About the Author

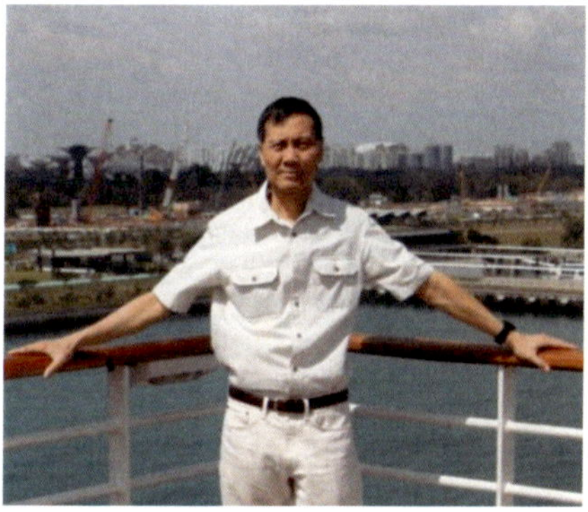

Dr. Lawrence S. Chan graduated from Massachusetts Institutes of Technology with double B.S. degrees in Life Sciences and Chemical Engineering. He subsequently attended University of Pennsylvania School of Medicine and received his M.D. degree there. After a fellowship in Biochemistry at the University of Pennsylvania Scheie Eye Institute, Dr. Chan completed an internship training at the Cooper Hospital/University Medical Center, and then obtained his residency training in Dermatology and a fellowship in Immunology at the University of Michigan Medical Center. After a short stint at the Wayne State University Medical School, Dr. Chan served as a junior faculty member at the Northwestern University for nine years, before he became an Associate Professor of Dermatology at the University of Illinois, College of Medicine in Chicago. Dr. Chan is a now a full Professor and the Department Head there. He has served as principle investigator of independent research grants supported by the Dermatology Foundation, Veterans Administration, and the National Institutes of Health. Dr. Chan has published two books, and over 30 book chapters, and more than 100 peer-reviewed biomedical articles.

Chapter 1

Historical Perspective

Most modern medical terminology is derived from either Latin or Greek, and most dermatology terms are no exception. The medical term "pemphigus" is in fact derived from the Greek word *pemphix*, translated into English as bubble, or blister. The term "vulgaris" is a Latin adjective, meaning common. Together, the term "pemphigus vulgaris" (PV) would indicate a common form of blistering skin disease. Although PV can be considered a common type of skin disorder of the blistering disease group and is the most prevalent form within the pemphigus group of disease (accounting for about 70% of patients affected by pemphigus), it is nevertheless a relatively rare skin disease. A major population-based study performed in the UK, however, showed an increasing trend in the development of PV, with an average annual increase of incidence at 11% over a study period of 10 years (1996 – 2006) (Langan et al. 2008).

The term "pemphigus" was first proposed by Boissier de Sauvages to classify an acute, febrile, blistering skin disease lasting two weeks in duration, probably similar to what we observe today as erythema multiforme (King and Holubar 1983). Wichmann first used the term "pemphigus" to describe a chronic form of blistering skin disease in 1791 (Jackson 1891, King and Holubar 1983). At that time, the diagnosis of "pemphigus" was based primarily on clinical observations, without the benefits of diagnostic clues derived from histological or immuno-microscopic tests. Naturally, blistering diseases with similar clinical morphology but distinct pathomechanism such as pemphigus foliaceus (PF) (Rock et al. 1990), dermatitis herpetiformis (Duhring 1983), bullous pemphigoid (BP) (Zillikens et al. 1997), epidermolysis bullosa acquisita (Gammon et al. 1982), and linear IgA bullous dermatosis (Zone et al. 1990), were possibly included in the diagnosis of "pemphigus" by physicians.

For a long period of time in history, PV was not distinguished from an equally common but less severe blistering skin disease now known as BP. Civatte is credited for the identification of pemphigus, and in certifying the presence of acantholytic epidermal cells, or the loss of cell-to-cell adhesion, in pemphigus. This critical finding provides a differentiating factor between pemphigus and other diseases where the blister occurred at the skin basement membrane level (i.e., intact epidermis without acantholysis) (Civatte 1943). Due to the subsequent histological findings of intra-epidermal blister and sub-epidermal blister, corresponding to PV and BP, respectively, a clear distinction between PV and BP was finally established. These tests also help distinguishing PV from other sub-epidermal blistering diseases (Lever 1951, 1953, Wilgram et al. 1961).

Before histological and immuno-microscopic techniques were available to provide a more accurate diagnosis for PV, physicians made the diagnosis based primarily on physical examination. One of the frequently used methods of clinical examination was to demonstrate a physical finding known as "Nikolskiy's sign," named after the late Russian physician Dr. Piotr Vasiliyevich Nikolskiy (Grando et al. 2003, Uzun and Durdu 2006). To demonstrate this sign, a physician gently pushes a blister with a finger from one side and look for the expansion of the blister border on the opposite side. The ability to induce the expansion was determined to be positive for Nikolskiy's sign, a finding supporting the diagnosis of PV (Uzun and Durdu 2006). Another physical finding that can be demonstrated in patients with PV is termed the "Asboe-Hansen sign." To demonstrate such a sign, the physician pushes down gently with a finger from the top of a blister and looks for peripheral expansion of the blister. The ability to expand the peripheral blister border is considered a positive "Asboe-Hansen sign," in support of a diagnosis of PV (Asboe-Hansen 1960, 1988). However, neither Nikolskiy's sign nor Asboe-Hansen sign is diagnostic for PV. They simply depict the loss of adherence of the epidermal cells. In addition to these two physical findings, one can demonstrate "acantholytic cells" by simply scraping a blister and examining the cells under a regular light microscope (Tzanck smear test). The presence of rounded, nucleated epidermal cells (acantholytic cells) supports the diagnosis of PV (Durdu et al. 2008). The possible reason for the positive Nikolskiy's and Asboe-Hansen signs in pemphigus and not in a disease like BP is the presence of acantholysis, an indication of severe loss of skin integrity, making it easier to expand the blister. In contrast, the absence of acantholysis in BP may preserve skin integrity to the extent that such expansion is not possible. Although these methods are no longer used commonly by physicians for the diagnosis of PV, it is interesting to note that a study published in 2006 demonstrated that Nikolskiy's sign does offer a moderately sensitive but highly specific tool for the diagnosis of pemphigus (Uzun and Durdu 2006).

Today, PV has been comprehensively characterized by medical science. We now recognize that it is an autoantibody-mediated intra-epidermal blistering disease affecting both mucous membranes and skin. Furthermore, the medical community has established solid diagnostic criteria, identified specific epidermal antigens targeted by the autoantibodies, and developed excellent therapeutic options for patients suffering from the disease. The progress for understanding and managing the disease notwithstanding, the disease still carries a mortality rate three times higher than the general population, according to one recent study (Langan et al. 2008). It will remain a high priority for the medical community to continue productive research toward greater understanding and refined management of the disease. In the following two chapters, the key developments regarding the diagnosis and treatment (Chapter 2) and the pathogenesis understanding (Chapter 3) will be discussed in greater detail.

Chapter 2

Key Developments in Diagnosis and Treatment

I. Histological Identification:

Historically, Civatte was the first to report the acantholytic epidermal cells that occurred in pemphigus (Civatte 1943). Lever was one of the first pathologists who clearly delineated the histopathological nature of PV, both at the light microscopic level and at the electron microscopic level (Lever 1951, 1953, and Wilgram et al. 1961). These findings delineated the blister-forming level as well as the nature of the blister in PV. Moreover, these findings also distinguished the intra-epithelial blister formation of PV from the sub-epithelial blister formation of BP and other sub-epithelial blistering diseases (Figure 1).

II. Immunofluorescence Microscopy:

The next key step in the delineation of diagnosis is the utilization of immunofluorescence microscopy. The importance of immunofluorescence microscopy in the diagnosis of PV is two-fold: First, it distinguishes PV as an immune-mediated skin disease rather than a heritable disease; second, it opens the door for a mechanistic approach to the treatment, that is, to utilize medications that have anti-inflammatory or immunosuppressive effects for the treatment. The identification of immune deposits by direct immunofluorescence microscopy (DIF), particularly immunoglobulin G (IgG) deposition at the cell surface of epidermis in peri-lesional skin specimen obtained from patients affected by PV, was a major step in making an accurate diagnosis of PV (Beutner et al. 1965) (Figure 2).

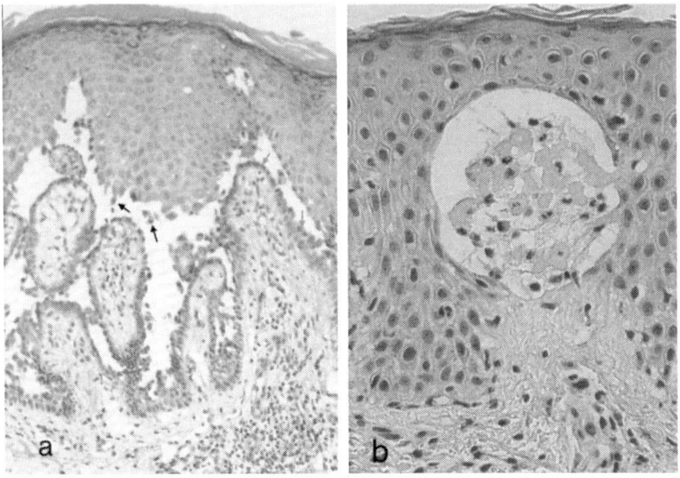

Figure 1. Histopathology of skin lesions obtained from patients affected by pemphigus vulgaris (a) contrasts with that from patients affected by bullous pemphigoid (b). Whereas the pemphigus vulgaris lesion is characterized by lower epidermis intra-epidermal blister and epidermal cell separation, or acantholysis (black arrows), and tomb stone pattern (blue arrows) (a), bullous pemphigoid lesion is typified by sub-epidermal blister with intact epidermis and eosinophil infiltration (blue arrows) (b).

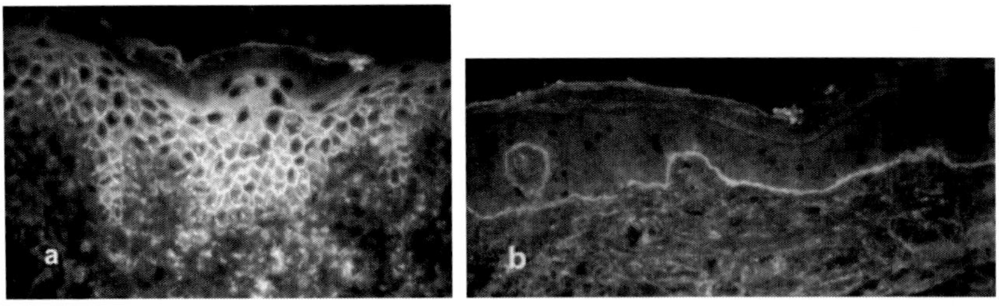

Figure 2. Direct immunofluorescence microscopy performed on a peri-lesional skin specimen obtained from patients of pemphigus vulgaris showing IgG deposits on the epidermal cell surface in a "chicken wiring" pattern (a), whereas a peri-lesional skin sample obtained from patients suffered from bullous pemphigoid had no epidermal cell surface deposits, but instead had a linear form of IgG deposits along the epidermal-dermal junction (b).

It also leads to the subsequent search for the source of immunological abnormality. The indirect immunofluorescence microscopy (IIF), which identifies patients' circulating autoantibodies of the IgG class that bind to the cell surface of the epithelial substrate, further helps confirm the diagnosis of PV by validating the serological origin of the IgG deposits at the patient's skin epidermis detected by DIF (Beutner and Jordon 1964, Beutner et al. 1965). After the IIF confirmation, the immunological nature of PV was then firmly established. Furthermore, these findings also pointed to a possible autoimmune nature of the disease, as such autoantibodies are now known to be present in patients' blood. What remained for physicians to determine in order to finally establish PV as an autoimmune disease was the ability to transfer the disease to an animal model (Rose and Bona 1993).

III. Systemic Corticosteroid:

Before the availability of systemic corticosteroid, most patients affected by PV succumbed to the disease due to water loss, electrolyte loss, and/or infection secondary to epidermis loss from the superficial blisters (Lever and White 1963). The available systemic corticosteroid has substantially reduced the mortality of PV (Lever & White 1963). However, the systemic steroid treatment created high morbidities due to its side effects of bone fracture, cataract, diabetes, mental changes, peptic ulcer, infections, and others (Lever and White 1963). The immunosuppressive medications were subsequently developed in part to act as a steroid-sparing agent (Lever and Schaumburg-Lever 1977, 1984).

IV. Immunosuppressives:

Developed to counter and reduce the steroid side effects on patients affected by immune-mediated diseases, immunosuppressives have been commonly utilized in helping these patients to control the disease. Azathioprine and mycophenolate mofetil have been used extensively and most commonly as potentially steroid-sparing medications, with azathioprine being an earlier treatment option (McMillan et al. 2015). Both medications seem to have equivalent efficacy in the treatment for PV (Beissert et al. 2006). Since mycophenolate mofetil became available and has been shown to have a lower tendency to cause liver toxicity (Beissert et al. 2007), it has become a more commonly used regimen among many physicians who take care of this group of patients. Mechanistically, both azathioprine and mycophenolate mofetil target the lymphocyte and act to suppress lymphocyte proliferation. However, unlike systemic corticosteroid, their actions in clinical improvement are not observed immediately. They may take between four and eight weeks for physicians to see the clinical effects. One of the major drawbacks in using these immunosuppressives is that they are not target-specific and they suppress the entire immune system or immune component regardless of the pathogenicity of the immune component. Thus, they would make PV patients receiving these medications more vulnerable to develop neoplasm or severe infection, at least on a theoretical basis. Although mycophenolate mofetil treatment in high doses — particularly in patients who received solid organ transplantation — has been associated with a small risk of internal malignancies, it has not shown such risk in a preliminary study of 139 patients treated for autoimmune blistering diseases by this medication, possibly due to the lower doses required to treat PV than that needed to prevent organ transplant rejection (Chan and Pappo 2013).

Azathioprine

As a precursor of active drug, azathioprine (AZA), once inside the human body, is converted to active medications of 6-mercaptopurine and 6-thioinosinic acid. These then act as DNA synthesis inhibitors for suppressing immune cells and keep them from proliferating, thus serving as a suppressor of immune function.

In a study enrolling 120 new patients of PV into one of four randomized treatment groups (prednisolone alone, prednisolone plus AZA, prednisolone plus mycophenolate mofetil, or prednisolone plus IV cyclophosphamide pulse) for one full year of follow up, the investigators found that the mean total of prednisolone used in the group of prednisolone alone was significantly higher than that in the other three groups (11.631 g vs 8.652 g). Furthermore, the mean dose of prednisolone used in the group that received prednisolone plus AZA (7.712 g) is significantly lower than that in the group that received prednisolone plus mycophenolate mofetil (9.798 g). However, it was not significantly lower than that in the group that received prednisolone plus cyclophosphamide (8.276 g), placing AZA as the most effective immunosuppressive in this study (Chams-Davatchi et al. 2007). In another retrospective study of 101 patients with a follow-up period of 7-21 years, different results were noted. Comparing four groups of patients of moderate to severe PV who received either 100 mg daily oral prednisone, prednisone plus 100 mg daily AZA, prednisone plus daily cyclosporine (2.5-3 mg/kg), or prednisone plus 100 mg daily cyclophosphamide, the investigators found that the corresponding average time for clinical remission was 33, 28, 30 and 23 months, respectively. This results in cyclophosphamide being the most effective in this study, although the addition of AZA was better than prednisone alone. Furthermore, the respective percent of patients remaining free of clinical relapse five years post-treatment were 55%, 50%, 43%, and 69%, again placing cyclophosphamide as the most effective medication in this respect (Olszewska et al. 2007). In a study published in 2011, a high dose of oral prednisone was compared with low dose prednisone combined with AZA in the treatment of PV patients. A group of 39 patients received either a daily high dose of prednisone (1.5 mg/kg) or a low alternate-day dose of prednisone combined with daily AZA. While both treatment regimens led to high rates of clinical responses, the mean prednisone dose required for complete remission and frequency of adverse events was significantly lower in the group that received combined medications. However, the mean time required to achieve complete remission was significantly higher for the same group as well (Chaidemenose et al. 2011). The most recent publication on randomized double-blind clinical trial of systemic corticosteroid with and without AZA in the treatment of PV was reported in 2013 (Chams-Davatchi, et al. 2013). In this study of 56 PV patients, the investigators found that AZA helped reduce prednisolone dose in the long run. Severe side effects encountered in patients treated with AZA include cholestatic hepatitis and life-threatening sepsis secondary to bone marrow suppression (Ben Salem et al. 2010, Tichy et al. 2014).

Mycophenolate Mofetil (MMF)

MMF's immunosuppressive function depends on its ability to inhibit DNA synthesis by targeting an important enzyme termed inosine monophosphate dehydrogenase. Its active metabolite, mycophenolic acid, impairs immune cell function.

A prospective, multicenter, randomized, nonblinded study comparing oral prednisolone plus either AZA or MMF on 33 PV patients and seven PF patients showed similar clinical efficacy with both medications. However, more patients treated with prednisolone plus AZA had experienced more grade

3 or 4 adverse effects (33% vs. 19%) (Beissert et al. 2006). Another study showed that MMF is a good corticosteroid-sparing agent, but it is not as effective as AZA (Chams-Davatchi et al. 2007). A 2010 report showed that MMF combined with systemic corticosteroids, in comparison to corticosteroid alone, proved beneficial in terms of secondary end points including time to response and duration of response. However, it did not show an advantage in a primary end point (percentage of patients responding to treatment with absence of new or persistent oral or skin lesions, and corticosteroid doses) (Beissert et al. 2010).

Cyclophosphamide

Cyclophosphamide (CYC) is another medication that could be used for PV treatment. As an immunosuppressive, CYC reduces immune response by suppressing cell proliferation, including immune cells. As a nitrogen mustard and an alkylating agent, CYC inhibits DNA synthesis on resting and proliferating cells, thus causing cell death.

Comparatively, the therapeutic effectiveness as well as toxicity index of CYC are in general higher than that of AZA and MMF. In some studies, CYC was utilized when AZA failed to achieve clinical remission and found it to be effective in bringing about remission (Ahmed and Hombal 1987). In one study of five PV patients, CYC in combination with prednisone was used as a first line of treatment, resulting in complete remission in all patients at follow up times from one to four years, with four of them requiring no medication (Fellner et al. 1978). Other investigators also reported success in treating two PV patients with a protocol combining low daily oral dose and high monthly intravenous (IV) pulse dose of CYC, resulting in clinical remission in seven to 10 months (Pandya and Sontheimer 1992). In a report from 2002, the investigators determined the long-term efficacy of a protocol including monthly IV pulse medications of dexamethasone (136 mg) for three consecutive days and CYC (500 mg) on the second day, with low daily dose of oral CYC (50 mg) on days between pulse treatments. This took place until partial remission, then continued with IV pulse and oral treatments for six months and one year, respectively. The investigators found that all 32 PV patients achieved complete clinical remission, with two to eight pulses required to reach partial remission and pulses ranging from eight to 32 to obtain complete remission. At the time of the report, all patients were in complete remission with a follow-up period of six months to 12 years (Kanwar et al. 2002). In the most recent study, a randomized, prospective, non-blinded clinical trial aiming to assess the efficacy of CYC pulse therapy as an adjuvant to oral corticosteroid for PV, investigators treated 60 patients with mild to moderate disease to received IV CYC and oral prednisone for one year, compared to oral prednisone alone. The result showed that CYC achieved improvements, though not statistically significant, on reduced time for clinical remission, higher portion achieved remission, lower relapse during treatment, and lower accumulative dose of systemic corticosteroids used (Sharma and Khandpur 2013). Reported serious adverse effects of CYC included hematuria, infection, and transitional cell carcinoma of the urinary bladder (Cummins et al. 2003). Close monitoring of side effects, particularly hematological and urological side effects, is needed in every patient receiving this medication (Cummins et al. 2003).

Methotrexate

Another immunosuppressive used in the treatment of PV is methotrexate (MTX), a known folate inhibitor (Baum et al. 2012, Tran et al. 2013). MTX inhibits key enzymes in folate metabolism, leading to inhibition of de novo purine synthesis, thus inhibiting DNA synthesis.

In a retrospective study of 30 patients of PV with a standard dose of 15 mg per week, 21 of 25 patients (84%) with moderate to severe disease scores improved at the six-month mark. Reduction of prednisone dose was achieved in 77% of treated patients, with statistically significant reduction of disease severity and prednisone dose (Baum et al. 2012). In another retrospective survey, 23 PV patients were examined for the steroid-sparing effectiveness of MTX, from data of patients who received the medication for a minimum of three consecutive months between 2000 and 2012 (Tran et al. 2013). In this survey, the investigators found that 91% of treated patients had clinical improvement, with 70% of patients achieving a prednisone-free state and a mean time of 18 months of remaining prednisone-free. In another 23% of patients, partial steroid-sparing effect was achieved with a mean daily dose of 6.75 mg prednisone for maintenance (Tran et al. 2013). Although it has been shown to be effective in these studies, MTX never became a mainstay of treatment likely due to its well-documented liver toxicity and the availability of other immunosuppressives. Nevertheless, it is an effective, readily available, and relatively inexpensive option for treating PV, provided careful monitoring of liver toxicity is regularly performed.

Cyclosporine

The potent effect of cyclosporine (CSP) is rested on its ability to block the gene transcription of many cytokines in activated T cells. CSP forms a complex with cyclophilin, which inhibits the phosphatase activity of calcineurin that regulates nuclear translocation on NFAT transcription factors (Matsuda and Koyasu 2000).

As an immunosuppressive commonly used in the prevention of solid organ transplant rejection, CSP also has been used in the treatment of PV (Barthelemy et al. 1988, Alijotas et al. 1990, Lapidoth et al. 1994, Mobini et al. 1997, Ioannides et al. 2000, Shivaswamy and Thappa 2007, Olszewska et al. 2007). While some investigators found that CSP was beneficial as a steroid-sparing agent for PV (Lapidoth et al. 1994, Mobini et al. 1997), others found that it was ineffective (Ioannides et al. 2000, Olszewska et al. 2007). Ironically, one patient actually developed PV after being treated with CSP for psoriasis (Caldarola et al. 2010). However, it is not clear in that case whether the medication is the cause of the PV development or the PV was developed as a result of "epitope spreading" secondary to the inflammatory injury occurred in psoriasis, as both PV and psoriasis can affect the same patient (Chan et al. 1998, Rallis et al. 2011). Other concerns are the developments of severe gingival hyperplasia, extensive keloid, and acute nephrotoxicity following CSP treatment in PV patients (Oettinger-Barak, et al. 2000, Mignogna et al. 2005, Shivaswamy and Thappa 2007).

V. Antibody Elimination Method:

When the use of standard immunosuppressives is limited by the presence of concomitant diseases or ineffectiveness, physical removal of patients' circulating antibodies may be one possible way to achieve clinical improvement. The German investigators reported a case of an elderly patient who was able to achieve autoantibody titer reduction parallel with complete clinical remission of disease after an initial series of weekly treatments, followed by monthly treatments of an adjuvant immunoadsorption therapy with the TheraSorb adsorber (Gunther et al. 2008). Others also reported successful immunoadsorption method, in combination with prednisone, in treating an adolescent patient of PV, also accompanying the autoantibody reduction (Ogata et al. 1999). Thus, the antibody elimination method can be considered when immunosuppressives are contraindicated. Physicians, however, should understand that this method is a temporary solution. The autoantibodies removed from the patients' circulation will be replaced by newly synthesized autoantibodies.

VI. Biologics

According to the US Food and Drug Administration, "Biological products include a wide range of products such as vaccines, blood and blood components, allergenics, somatic cells, gene therapy, tissues, and recombinant therapeutic proteins. Biologics can be composed of sugars, proteins, or nucleic acids or complex combinations of these substances, or may be living entities such as cells and tissues. Biologics are isolated from a variety of natural sources — human, animal, or microorganism — and may be produced by biotechnology methods and other cutting-edge technologies. Gene-based and cellular biologics, for example, often are at the forefront of biomedical research, and may be used to treat a variety of medical conditions for which no other treatments are available" (FDA).

Intravenous Immunoglobulin

Intravenous immunoglobulin (IVIg) treatment, one of the early biologics for PV, has also been reported to be beneficial for this group of patients, although its mechanism for improving PV condition is not clearly defined (Bewley and Keefe 1996, Bystryn and Jiao 2006). In IVIg treatment, serum-derived and infection-eliminated immunoglobulin from healthy individuals is administered into the PV patients by IV infusion. In a relatively large study, 12 patients with severely active PV, unresponsive to conventional therapy of high doses of systemic corticosteroids with or without cytotoxic drugs, were treated with a single dose of IVIg (400 mg/kg/day for five days), with concurrent immunosuppressives (CYC or AZA). The investigators found that within one week of IVIg initiation, PV lesions were controlled in most patients and by week 3 the average corticosteroid doses were reduced by 40%. In addition, circulating autoantibodies to epidermal cell surface by IIF were lessened on the average 59% in week 1 and 70% by week 2 of IVIg initiation. Interestingly, the reduction of PV autoantibodies was selective, as antibody levels to varicella-herpes zoster remained the same in four patients they measured. However, it is not clear whether these antibodies to herpes virus the investigators measured were in part from the IVIg the patients received (Bystryn and Jiao 2006). Side effects of IVIg that have been reported included deep venous thrombosis, pulmonary embolism, and myocardial infarction. Thus, history of coronary artery disease, immobility, hypertension or risk factors for thrombotic complications would be considered as relative contraindications to IVIg therapy (Sheehan and Lesher 2004).

Rituximab

Rituximab (RTX), a humanized antibody, targets B cells (anti-CD20) by mechanisms of direct signaling for apoptosis induction, complement-dependent cytotoxicity, and antibody-dependent cellular cytotoxicity (Weiner 2010).

Along with humanized antibodies developed to treat other immune-mediated skin diseases like psoriasis, biologics have also been in the forefront of treatment for PV in the last 10 years. Since PV is directly mediated by autoantibodies, which is a product of B-lymphocytes, an antibody directly targeting these white cells became an obvious choice of medication development. An antibody developed to target B-lymphocytes in an intermediate stage of maturity, specifically on its unique surface marker CD20, RTX, has been examined in many patients affected by PV over the last few years (Ahmed et al. 2006, Peterson and Chan 2009, Balighi et al. 2013, Colliou et al. 2013, Cho et al. 2014, Ellebrecht et al. 2014, Gregorious et al. 2014, Heelan et al. 2014, Kanwar et al. 2014, Leshem et al. 2014, Vinay et al. 2014, Ahmed and Shetty 2015, Amber and Hertl 2015, Ingen-Housz-Oro et al. 2015).

In their 2006 report, Ahmed reported a study of 11 PV patients who failed to achieve complete remission with conventional therapy and had 30% or greater body surface areas affected, three more mucous membranes involved, or both. After receiving two monthly cycles of three weekly RTX (375 mg/square meter body surface area) and one weekly IVIg (2 gram/kg body weight), followed by four more monthly cycles of one each of RTX and IVIg, the investigators found that nine of these patients had rapid resolution of their skin diseases and were able to achieve clinical remission for the duration ranging from 22 to 37 months. The investigators were also able to taper off all immunosuppressives and corticosteroid from the patients before the six-month treatment time frame (Ahmed et al. 2006). Interestingly, all circulating B-lymphocytes were undetectable shortly after initial RTX dose but subsequently returned (Ahmed et al. 2006).

A 2012 review of RTX treatment for a total of 272 PV patients in 42 studies published between 2000 and 2012 shed some light on the overall outcome of RTX therapy (Zakka et al. 2012). Comparing two distinct protocols, the lymphoma protocol (which consists of four weekly infusions of RTX at a dose of 375 mg/square meter body surface) and the rheumatoid arthritis protocol (which consists of one gram RTX on day 1 and day 15 of the month), the authors found that while both protocols were effective in treating recalcitrant PV, the lymphoma protocol resulted in a lower response rate, relapse rate, and serious infection, but higher mortality and some non-responders. On the other hand, the rheumatoid arthritis protocol showed a higher response rate, relapse rate, and infection, but lower mortality and no non-responders (Zakka et al. 2012). While preliminary clinical remission was achieved in 90-95% of patients within six weeks, complete remission occurred later between three and four months. In addition, the majority of the patients with complete remission were still on lower dose of medications (systemic corticosteroids and immunosuppressives). The physicians in the field, however, were concerned about the high infection/septicemia rate occurring in both protocols, while they recognized RTX as the best currently available biologic for PV (Zakka et al. 2012, Shetty and Ahmed 2013, Ahmed and Shetty 2015).

In a 2014 report, a modified fixed dose RTX originally developed for rheumatoid arthritis treatment was found to be very good in controlling PV (Heelan et al. 2014). This protocol consists of giving intravenous RTX one gram on day 1 and day 15, followed by 500 mg of the same medication every six months as clinically indicated. The investigators reported that all patients improved on this protocol, that 89% of patients obtained complete remission with 61% and 28% off and on adjuvant treatment at the time of remission, respectively. The report indicated that the medium time for relapse was 15 months from the initial treatment cycle (Heelan et al. 2014).

Although some successes have been documented in the literature on the management of PV, one needs to be cautious about the long-term effectiveness of anti-CD20 antibodies. As this biologic is a humanized antibody, the small amount of animal protein contained inside the anti-CD20 antibody may

IV. Epitope Spreading as a Mechanism of Disease Progression:

An "epitope" is a stretch of a biological molecule (most likely a protein) with a molecular size of 1 kilo Dalton or larger. Epitope is formed in a way that can evoke an immune response by a T cell or antibody and it tends to become the target of autoimmune reaction. It is also called "antigenic determinant." "Epitope spreading" describes an immunological phenomenon in which an inflammatory or autoimmune event results in tissue damage, leading to exposing previously unrecognized or hidden antigenic epitope to autoreactive lymphocytes, ultimately inducing an autoimmune reaction to the newly exposed antigenic epitope (Chan et al. 1998) (Figure 4).

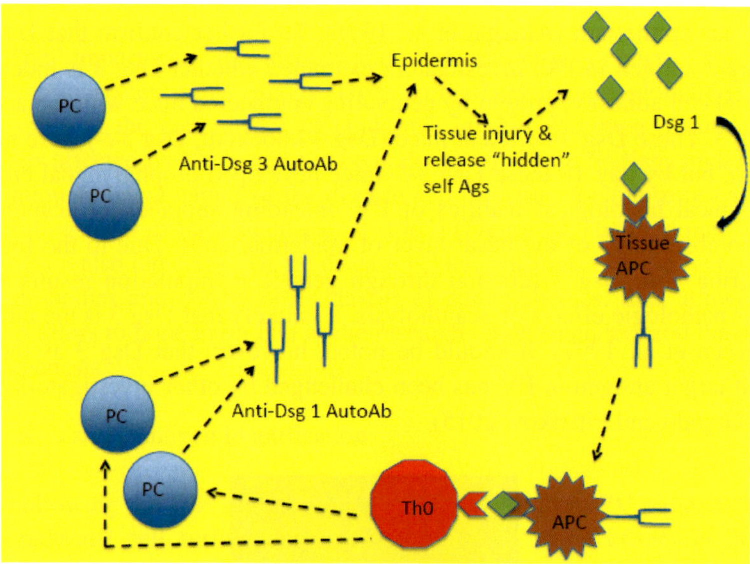

Figure 4. Schematic diagram demonstrates the concept of immunological phenomenon "epitope spreading" in pemphigus vulgaris. The process starts with an initial autoimmune event, with Dsg 3 autoantibodies causes oral mucosal epithelial tissue damage, exposing some previously "hidden" antigenic determinant (epitope, Dsg 1) to tissue antigen presenting cells that were attracted to the damaged site by chemokines. The subsequent interaction between the antigen presenting cells and helper T cells then leads to proliferation of these T cells, and the T cells-B cells interaction that follows would trigger the production of autoantibody against this antigenic determinant, i.e., epitope (Dsg 1), resulting in the expansion of disease to involve skin. AutoAb, autoantibodies; PC, plasma cells, Th0, helper T Cells, APC, antigen presenting cells; Ags, antigens; Dsg, desmoglein; AutoAb, autoantibodies.

The newly recognized epitope that is exposed can be within the same protein (intra-molecular epitope spreading) or a different protein (inter-molecular epitope spreading) (Chan et al. 1998, Salato et al. 2005, Pigozzi et al. 2008). In PV, this immune phenomenon has been documented in some patients (Salato et al. 2005, Pigozzi et al. 2008). In one study, investigators followed the serology of patients who initially developed lesions exclusively on oral mucosae and then developed generalized skin lesions. They found that only anti-Dsg 3 autoantibodies were present when the lesions were restricted within the oral cavity and that both anti-Dsg 3 and anti-Dsg 1 autoantibodies were detected when the lesions were expanded to affect skin areas (Ding et al. 1997). Thus, the inter-molecular epitope spreading may play a role here with this possible scenario: The targeting of Dsg 3 by autoantibodies induce mucosal epithelial cell acantholysis, this cell-cell separation opens up other antigen such as Dsg 1 to be exposed to antigen-presenting cells that came through the inflamed site, leading to activation of autoreactive T cells, T cell-B cell interaction, and then autoreactive B cell activation, eventually resulting in autoantibody production against Dsg 1, which will subsequently be responsible for inducing blisters of the skin areas (Figure 4).

V. Animal Modeling: Passive Transfer of Disease

Anhalt et al. was the first group of investigators who proved that, by passively transferring serum IgG from patients affected by PV to newborn mice, a skin manifestation similar to that of human PV patients can be induced, with resulting clinical blisters and erosions, as well as histologic, ultrastructural, and immunofluorescence features of PV, firmly defining PV as an autoimmune disease (Rose and Bona 1993). In addition, the titer of these serum IgGs correlated with the extent of induced clinical blisters and erosions, further supporting the role of these IgG antibodies in the blister formation (Anhalt et al. 1982). Subsequently, other investigators determined that purified autoantibodies from PV patients that are specific for Dsg 3, when passively transferred to newborn mice, induced oral mucosal blisters specifically, further confirming the role of autoantibodies to Dsg 3 in the PV pathogenesis (Culton et al. 2015).

VI. Animal Modeling: Active Induction of Disease

Demonstration of an actively induced disease is the final and most important step in understanding the pathomechanism of PV. Toward this end,

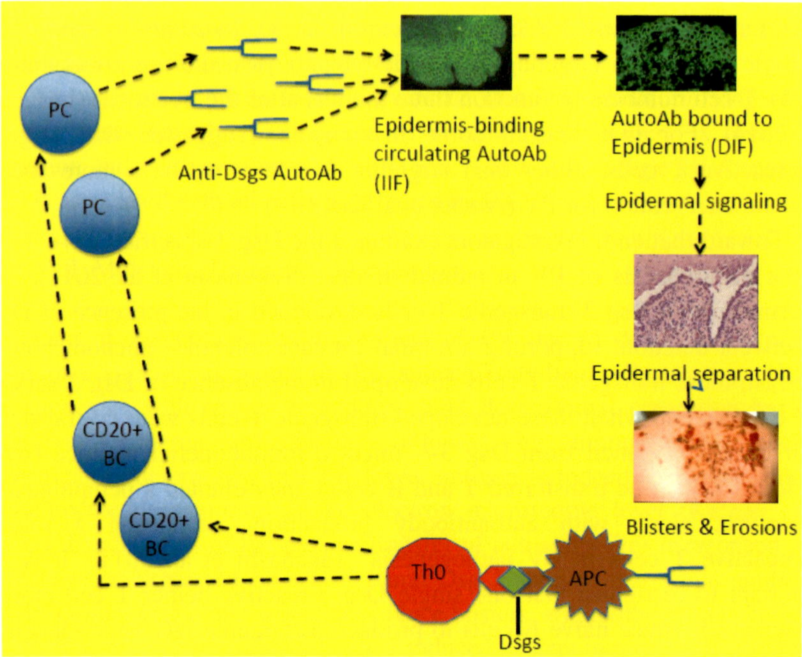

Figure 5. Schematic diagram depicting our current understanding of the pathophysiology of PV. The process starts with antigen presentation of Dsgs to helper T cells, leading to autoreaction of T cells. The subsequent T cell-B cell interaction then results in autoantibodies production against Dsgs. The circulating epidermis-binding autoantibodies (as detected by IIF) eventually bind to the epidermal cell surface of patients' skin (as illustrated by DIF), resulting in epidermal signaling, leading to epidermal separation (as determined by histology), with the final clinical outcome of blisters and erosions. APC, antigen presenting cells, Th0, helper T cells; BC, B cells; PC, plasma cells; Dsgs, desmogleins; AutoAb, autoantibodies. Black dash arrows denote direction of immunological progression.

In summary, a schematic diagram depicting our current understanding of pathophysiology of PV is illustrated in Figure 5.

Chapter 4

Clinical Manifestations

I. Epidemiology:

Data gathered from epidemiological studies around the globe provided physicians with a comprehensive picture of the age of onset, gender, and other factors associated with PV. In South Africa, a study published in 2001 revealed PV being much less common than PF, with a mean age of onset of 48 years and a female to male ratio of 1.7 to 1 (Aboobaker et al. 2001). In the United Kingdom, PV was determined to be much less common than bullous pemphigoid, with an incidence rate of 7 per 1 million person years, a female to male ratio of 1.94 to 1, a median age of onset of 71 years, and an overall mortality rate 3.3 times that of the general population (Langan et al. 2008). In Northwestern Romania, PV was reported to be the most common autoimmune blistering disease at 58%, with an incidence of 4 per 1 million per year and an average onset age of 53 years (Baican et al. 2010). In Thailand, a survey of 124 pemphigus patients revealed that PV is the most common subtype (79%), that the mean age of onset for PV is 45 years, and that the female to male ratio is 2:1 (Kulthanan et al. 2011). An epidemiological survey for PV patients in Western Turkey showed that the mean age of onset was 48 years, the female to male ratio was 1.64 to 1, and that PV was the most common clinical subtype in that region (Bozdaq and Bilqin 2012). In Taiwan, a nationwide population-based study of 853 PV patients between 2002 and 2009 showed that the incidence of PV in Taiwan was 4.7 per million per year, that the mean age of onset was 52 years, that the female to male ratio was 1.33 to 1, and that the overall mortality rate of PV patients was more than twice that of the general population (Huang et al. 2012). In a recent publication based on a 10-year retrospective study of the Northwest Chinese population, ~~the~~ investigators determined from a total of 221 PV patients that the mean age of onset was 44 years, that female to male ratio was 1.40 to 1, and that 56% of patients had both mucosal and skin diseases (Zhu et al. 2014). To summarize, from a global perspective, PV seems to have an incidence ranging from 4 to 7 per million per year, with a higher female to male ratio (ranging from 1.33:1 to 2:1), and an average age of onset ranging from 44 to 71. The overall mortality rate of PV patients is approximately 2 to 3 times higher than that of the general population.

II. Mucous membrane involvement:

By various reports, a majority of patients who had PV with both skin and mucosa involvements developed clinical manifestations in oral mucosae first, with mucosal lesions preceding the skin lesions. In some patients, the skin lesions and oral lesions surfaced simultaneously. In other patients, the oral lesions remained the only manifestation without any apparent skin involvement. For the patients who had lesions restricted to oral mucosae, it is not clear whether the progression to involve skin was suppressed by treatments prescribed for the oral lesion (thus preventing "epitope spreading") or the progression was somehow pre-determined to be restricted to the oral mucosae.

Oral lesions manifest rarely as small blisters and more commonly as erosions (Figure 6). In one survey, the most commonly observed oral lesions of PV were buccal mucosa (90%), posterior wall of pharynx (67.5%), and upper epiglottis (85%). In addition, the nasal vestibule was affected in 70% of patients (Fernandez et al. 2012). Lip, tongue, and the floor of the mouth can also be involved with erosions or ulcerations (Munhoz et al. 2011, Nguyen and Ahmed 2014). The types of oral mucosal lesions include clear fluid-filled blisters (rare), erythema (Figure 6d), erosions (Figure 6b, 6c, 6f), crusted lesions (Figure 6e), and membrane-covered bullae (Figure 6a, 6c).

In theory, any mucous membranes that are squamous epithelium in nature can be affected in patients with PV. However, oral mucosa is primarily affected clinically. Some of the less commonly affected mucous membrane areas include conjunctivae (Hodak et al. 1990, Uludag et al. 2013), esophagus (Amichai et al. 1996, Khamaysi and Eliakim 2008, Asarch et al. 2012), penis (Stieger et al. 2013), perianal (Figure 7a), vagina (Figure 7b), and perineum (Patsatsi et al. 2009).

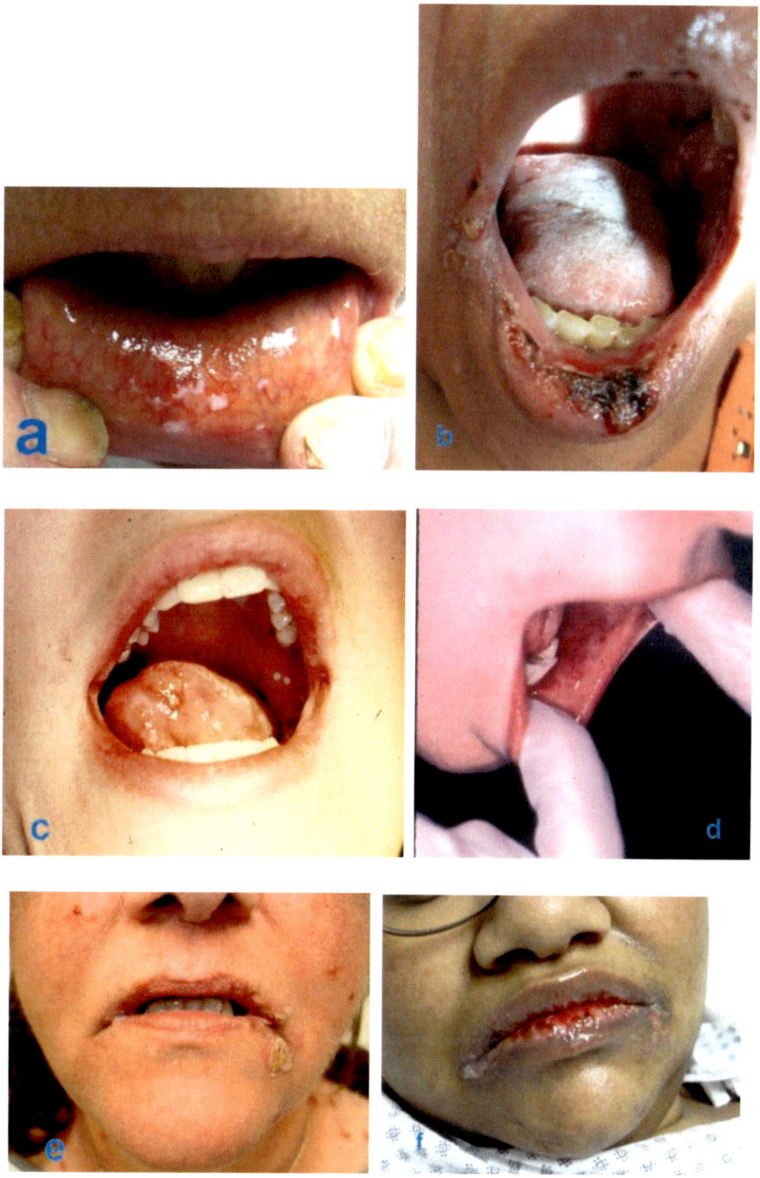

Figure 6. Various manifestations of oral mucosal lesions of pemphigus vulgaris.

Surprisingly, one study found that active laryngeal lesions (ulcers or blisters) were present in 40% of PV patients (16/40 PV patients), with low-grade lesions being more common (Mahmoud et al. 2012). Since this data represents statistics from one region of the world, more studies, particularly from other parts of the world, will help in confirming the universal presence of this finding. In one reported case, laryngeal lesion was the only clinical manifestation with clinical symptoms of hoarseness, hemoptysis, and dysphagia (Vasiliou et al. 2007).

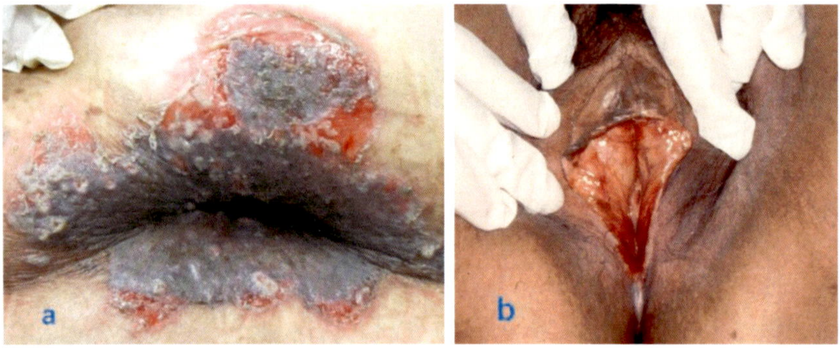

Figure 7. Other mucosal lesions of pemphigus vulgaris.

Thus, when clinicians encounter PV patients, it will be appropriate to inquire about symptoms and signs of disease manifestations in all mucosal membranes to ensure no areas of involvement are missed. A simple inquiry about eye irritation, epistaxis, dysphagia, hoarseness, dysuria and pain on defecation will cover potential involvement of conjunctivae, nasal mucosae, esophagus, larynx, genitaria and perianal areas, respectively.

III. Skin involvement:

On the skin (Figure 8), lesions are usually manifested as crusted papules (Figure 8f, 8g, 8h, 8i), erythema (Figure 8a, 8c), flaccid fluid-filled bullae (Figure 8d) and erosions (Figure 8b, 8c, 8d, 8e). Since the flaccid bullae break easily, many patients initially present their diseases as diffuse erosions (Figure 8b), without any observable blisters.

Any areas of the skin can be involved. However, the severity of the skin involvement varies from patient to patient. Some studies have indicated that the extent of skin affected is correlated to the titer of the circulating autoantibodies detected in a given patient and this clinical finding is supported by passive transfer animal model study (Anhalt et al. 1982). This antibody titer–skin extent correlation makes good clinical sense, as more serum autoantibody available to circulate to the skin and to bind to the skin target antigen Dsg 3, the larger amount of skin that may be induced to blisters.

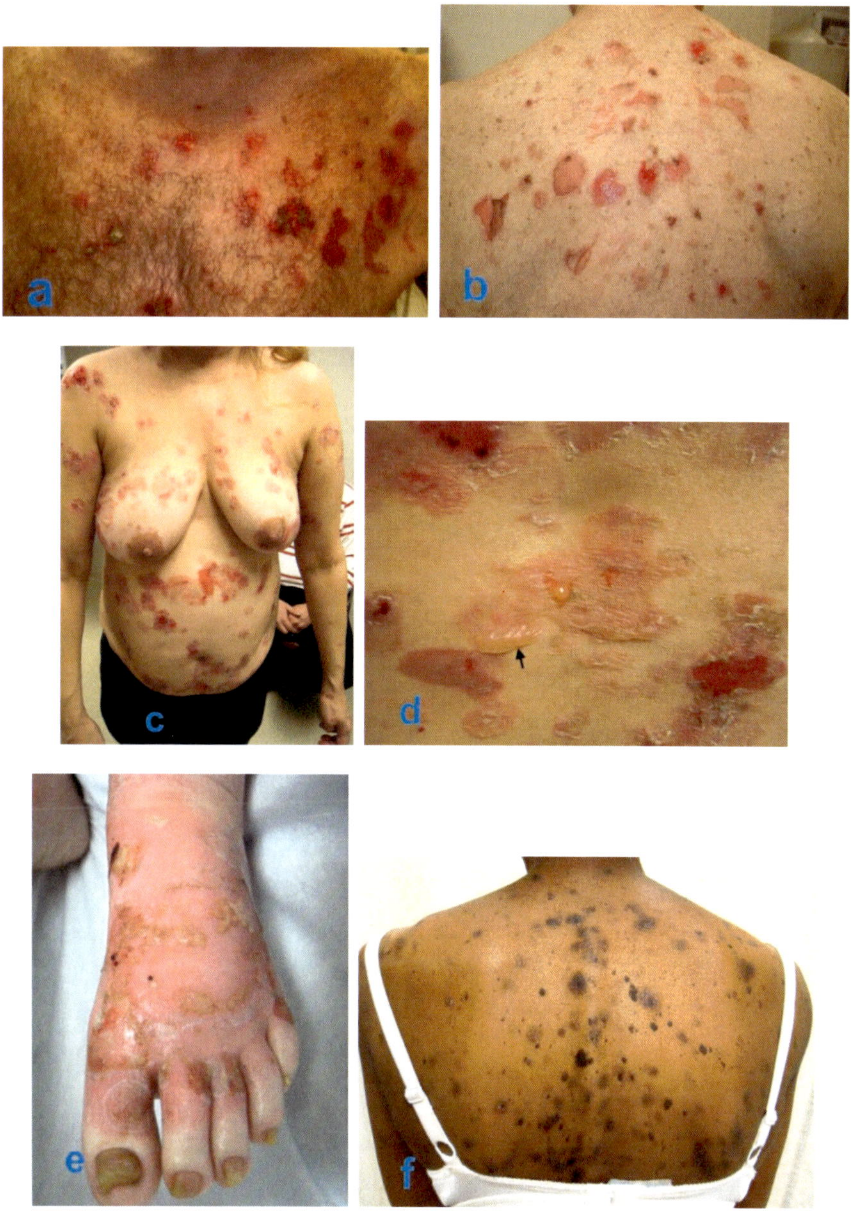

Figure 8. (Continued)

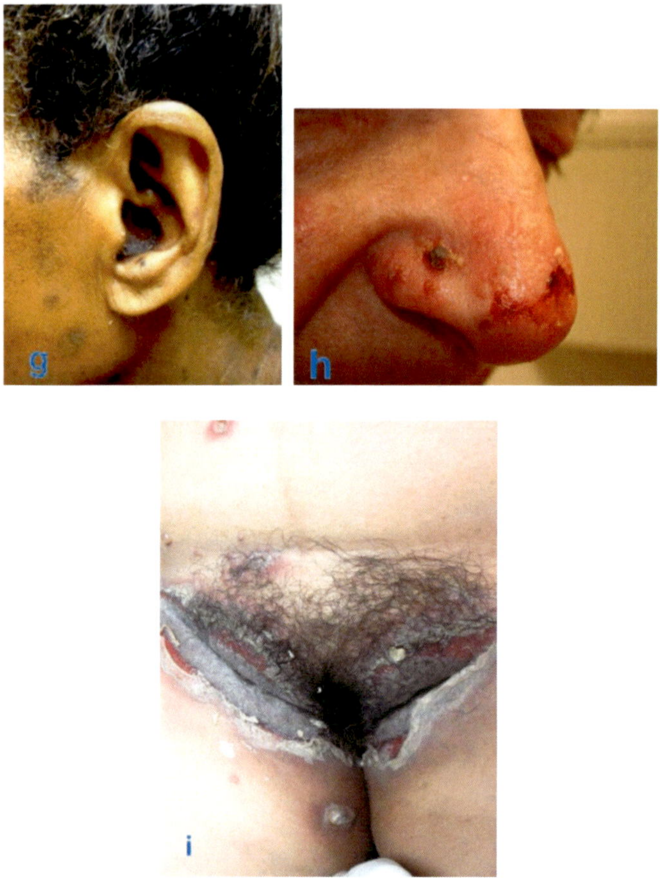

Figure 8. Various manifestations of skin lesions of pemphigus vulgaris.

The scalp can be affected in patients affected by PV (Figure 9). In some patients, their scalp lesions, usually manifested as crusted inflamed lesions with alopecia, became the most difficult to treat (Patsatsi et al. 2009, Kamphausen et al. 2012). Hair follicle acantholysis has been documented histologically. Hair loss (alopecia) has been identified as an unusual manifestation of PV (Hadayer et al. 2013, Veraitch et al. 2013). The identification of a novel Dsg protein, Dsg 4, responsible for hair growth and the presence of anti-Dsg 4 autoantibodies in some patients affected by PV strongly support a notion that anti-Dsg 4 autoantibodies may be responsible for the alopecia in these PV patients (Kljuic et al. 2003). Nevertheless, it remains to be sorted out whether the presence of anti-Dsg 4 autoantibodies are detected only in the PV patients with alopecia or scalp lesions, and not present in those PV patients without alopecia or scalp lesions.

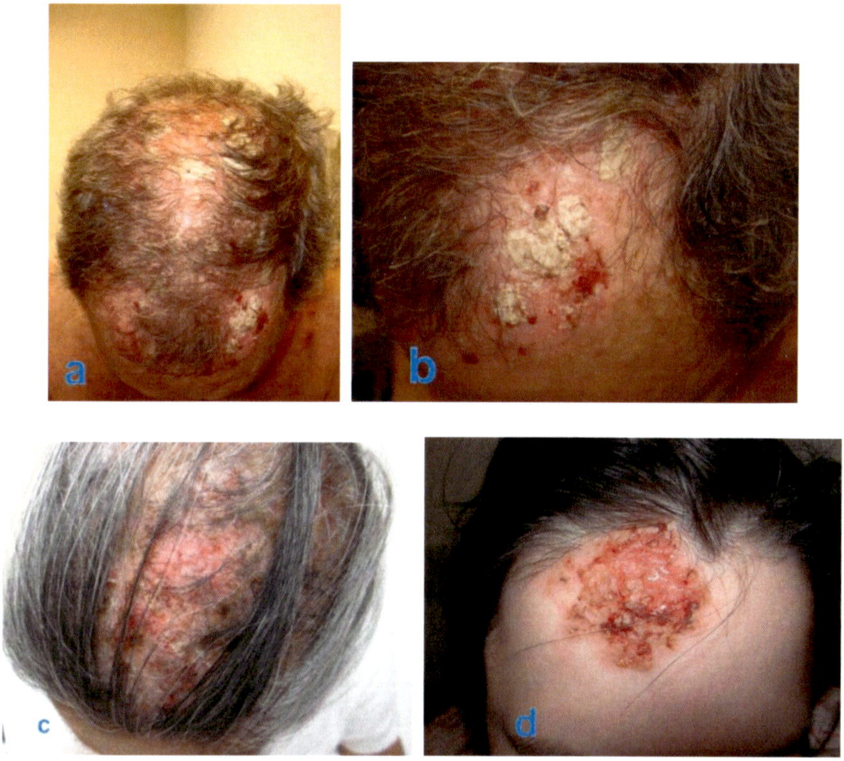

Figure 9. Scalp lesions of pemphigus vulgaris manifested clinically (a, b, c, d) with acantholysis of hair follicles documented in histology.

Nail involvement is one of the rare observations in PV. However, one PV patient was reported to have 19 nails affected, manifested with severe nail fold inflammation, hemorrhagic paronychia and subungual hemorrhage (Patsatsi et al. 2009).

Are there factors contributing to the prognosis of PV disease? One study looked into 95 patients affected by pemphigus (79 had PV and 16 had PF) and determined that patients of Indo-Asian origin (compared to white patients), a younger age at onset (40 years), and higher initial autoantibody titers (by IIF on normal human skin substrate) had a significantly longer duration of the disease (Saha et al. 2014).

Chapter 5

Clinical Variants

There are several clinical variants of the classic manifestations of pemphigus vulgaris: Drug-induced PV, pemphigus vegetans, paraneoplastic pemphigus and IgA pemphigus. These diseases could be classified as PV variants because they are clinically similar to PV and the patients have autoantibodies to Dsg 3, the PV antigen.

I. Drug-induced PV

Like some other skin eruption caused by medications, drugs have been identified as an inducer or trigger for the development of a blistering disease sharing substantial clinical, histopathological, and immunological features of classic PV (Wilson et al. 1986, Korman et al. 1991, Brenner et al. 1997, Landau and Brenner 1997, Feng et al. 2011, Baroni et al. 2012, Gholizadeh et al. 2012, Yoshimura et al. 2014). Drugs that have been reported to induce PV include thiol-containing medications (captopril, d-penicillamine), amoxicillin/clavulanic acid, and cefadroxil. Consistent with a PV variant, autoantibodies from the serum of these patients recognized the classic PV antigen (Korman et al. 1991, Brenner et al. 1997). Histopathology finding of a drug-induced PV is no different from that of a classic PV and therefore cannot be used to distinguish drug-induced PV from classic PV. Thus, a detailed clinical history will be important to sort out the drug-induced cases from the classic cases (Landau and Brenner 1997). Most patients responded very well with withdrawal of the offending medications and conventional treatments for

PV, though some cases became chronic and protracted diseases (Yoshimura et al. 2014).

II. Pemphigus vegetans

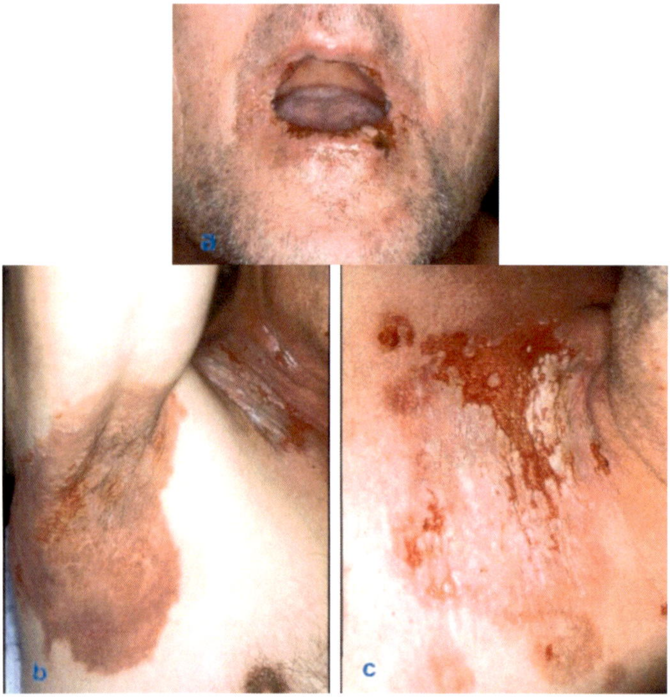

Figure 10. Clinical features of pemphigus vegetans.

Whether pemphigus vegetans is a unique clinical variant of PV or a clinical spectrum of PV is not yet settled. In either case, the vegetans form of pemphigus has a distinct clinical presentation that the lesions, primarily on mouth and skin folds (intertriginous areas), somehow became exophytic with the appearance of vegetation or pustules, thus the development of the medical term "pemphigus vegetans" (Figure 10). The clinical uniqueness of pemphigus vegetans notwithstanding, studies have confirmed that the autoantibodies from this group of patients also target the autoantigens documented in patients with PV, i.e., Dsg 3 (Hashizume et al. 1993, Ohata et al. 1996). In some patients, autoantibodies against desmocollins and plakins were observed (Hashimoto et al. 1994, Cozzani et al. 2007, Saruta et al. 2013). Histologically, pemphigus vegetans lesion has some features distinct from the classic PV, including prominent infiltration of neutrophils and eosinophils (Hashizume et al. 1993). A clear logical explanation as to why the identical autoantibodies would eventually lead to two distinct clinical morphologies, supported by solid scientific data, is not yet available. But such information will be useful for physicians to understand and perhaps helpful for treatment, as well. Treatments for pemphigus vegetans, in general, are similar to those used for PV.

III. Paraneoplastic pemphigus (PNP)

Although clinical cases similar to PNP were known for some time, Grant Anhalt was the first investigator who provided strong scientific evidence linking this clinical variant with concomitant neoplasm and coined the term PNP (Anhalt, et al. 1990). In this first series of patient cases, Anhalt et al. have demonstrated a rather unique set of clinical manifestations of PNP, including particularly severe hemorrhagic stomatitis, involvement of multiple mucous membranes, possible life-threatening pulmonary involvement, strong resistance to conventional immunosuppressive therapies, and high mortality rate (Anhalt 1997, 2004). The most commonly observed clinical feature is painful and persistent stomatitis, manifested as ulcerations and erosions of any oropharynx with visible epithelial necrosis and lichenoid morphology and involvement of vermilion of the lips (Figure 11). In addition, the lateral tongue is also affected with severe pain. The morphology of skin lesions are more variable, ranging from toxic epidermal necrolysis (TEN)-like large confluent erosions, PV-like flaccid blisters and erosions, bullous pemphigoid-like tense bullae, erythema multiforme-like erythema surrounded bullae, Graft-versus-host disease-like dermatitis, to lichen planus-like lichenoid dermatitis (Anhalt 2004, Czernik et al. 2011, Frew and Murrell 2011) (Figure 12). Other mucous membranes can also be affected and nail involvement can be very severe (Figure 13). A very serious extra-cutaneous involvement of PNP is the life-threatening pulmonary disease called "bronchiolitis obliterans," documented by the IgG immune deposition at the bronchial epithelium (Fullerton et al. 1992, Hoffman et al. 2003). Furthermore, IgG was also found to deposit in kidney, urinary bladder, and muscles as well (Nguyen et al. 2001). CD8+ (cytotoxic subset) T cells are suggested to be involved in this highly fatal disease (Nguyen et al. 2001, Hoffman et al. 2003). In addition to sharing some clinical features with the classic PV, some patients affected by PNP also had lichenoid dermatitis, and in some cases lichenoid dermatitis precedes the clinical manifestation of blisters, raising the possible role of "epitope spreading" in the disease progression (Bowen et al. 2000, Chan 2000). In most cases, a definite internal neoplasm is identified. The various neoplasms associated with PNP, in–descending order of frequency, are non-Hodgkin's lymphoma (NHL) (42%), chronic lymphocytic lymphoma (CLL) (29%), Cattleman's tumor (10%), thymoma (6%), sarcoma (6%) and Waldenstrom's macroglobulinemia (6%) (Anhalt 2004). On the histopathological ground, PNP lesions have somewhat unique characteristics when compared to PV, with several major distinct features like vacuolar change of the basilar epidermis, dyskeratotic keratinocytes, and epidermal exocytosis of inflammatory cells, as well as common features of PV of suprabasal cleft formation and acantholytic keratinocytes (Horn and Anhalt 1992). In some cases, significant lichenoid dermatitis pattern, with a "band-like" lymphocytes infiltration along the epidermal-dermal junction and keratinocyte necrosis, is observed (Anhalt 2004) (Figure 14). In other cases, the evidence of flank acantholysis, the typical histologic feature of PV, cannot be found (Anhalt 2004). Similarly, the immunopathology findings in PNP by DIF also showed uniqueness when compared to PV. In addition to the "chicken wiring" pattern of IgG deposition, some cases of PNP showed IgG deposition along the epidermal-dermal junction, a finding similar to that of "pemphigus erythematosus," a disease that combines the presentation of pemphigus and lupus erythematosus (Anhalt et a. 1990, Anhalt 2004) (Figure 14). Most patients also have IgG circulating autoantibodies binding to the transitional epithelium substrate like rat bladder by IIF (Anhalt et al. 1990) (Figure 14). The evidence linking PNP with PV, in addition to the clinical morphology similarity, is that patients with PNP developed circulating autoantibodies to the epidermal adhering protein Dsg 3 (the PV antigen), just like patients affected by PV. Additionally, these autoantibodies to Dsg 3 are pathogenic in inducing blisters in newborn mice (Amagai et al. 1998). Therefore PNP could be classified as a variant of PV. Physicians should recognize that children can be affected by PNP predominantly associated with Cattleman's disease as well as fatality primarily due to bronchiolitis obliterans (Mimouni et al. 2002, Lane et al. 2004, Daneshpazhooh et al. 2012). Autoantibodies from PNP patients also recognized several epithelial proteins of the plakin family: envoplakin, periplakin, and desmoplakin (Oursler et al. 1992, Anhalt 2004). Due to the involvement of internal organs, a term "paraneoplastic autoimmune multiorgan syndrome" has been used in parallel with PNP (Nguyen et al. 2001, Czernik et al. 2011). The diagnosis of PNP is based on severe and distinct clinical features, particularly painful stomatitis; histological findings of lichenoid changes, acantholysis, and necrotic keratinocytes; and immunopathology of IgG deposits to epithelial cell surface (sometimes also to basement membrane) and IgG circulating autoantibodies to rat bladder (Anhalt 2004). A study of 29 PNP sera, published in 1995, reported that murine urinary bladder used as a substrate to test for PNP autoantibody gave a sensitivity of 75% and a specificity of 83%, adequate as a good screening test. However, investigators urged that a test for identification of PNP-specific antigens (plakins) be performed as well (Helou et al. 1995). Physicians also need to recognize that a false negative DIF finding is frequent and repeated study on a different site may be needed (Anhalt 2004). Regarding treatment, complete surgical removal of primary neoplasm would be preferred. Interestingly, rituximab has been shown to be effective in controlling some cases of non-Hodgkin's lymphoma-associated PNP, which tends to be resistant to most conventional therapy (Heizmann et al. 2001, Barnadas, et al. 2006).

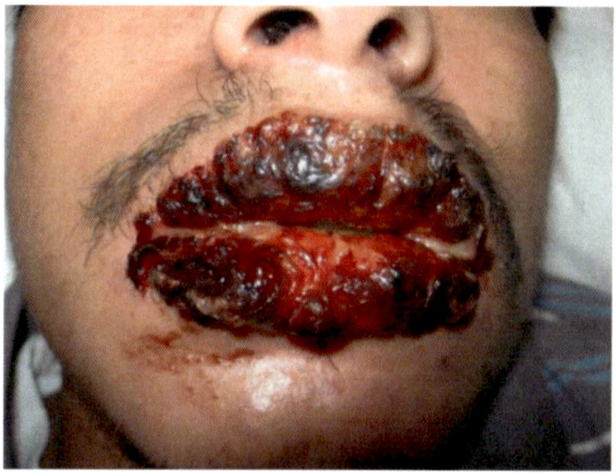

Figure 11. Painful and persistent stomatitis is a characteristic feature of paraneoplastic pemphigus.

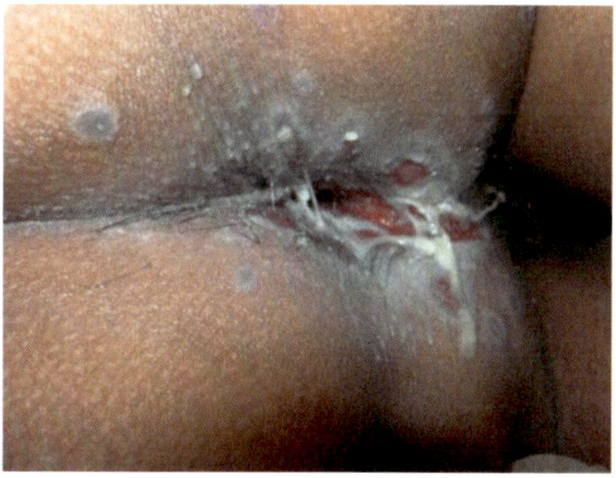

Figure 12. Manifestations of peri-rectal lesions in paraneoplastic pemphigus.

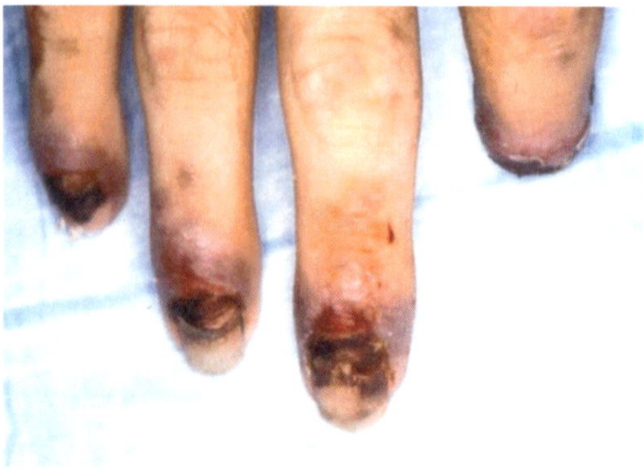

Figure 13. Manifestations of nail lesions in paraneoplastic pemphigus.

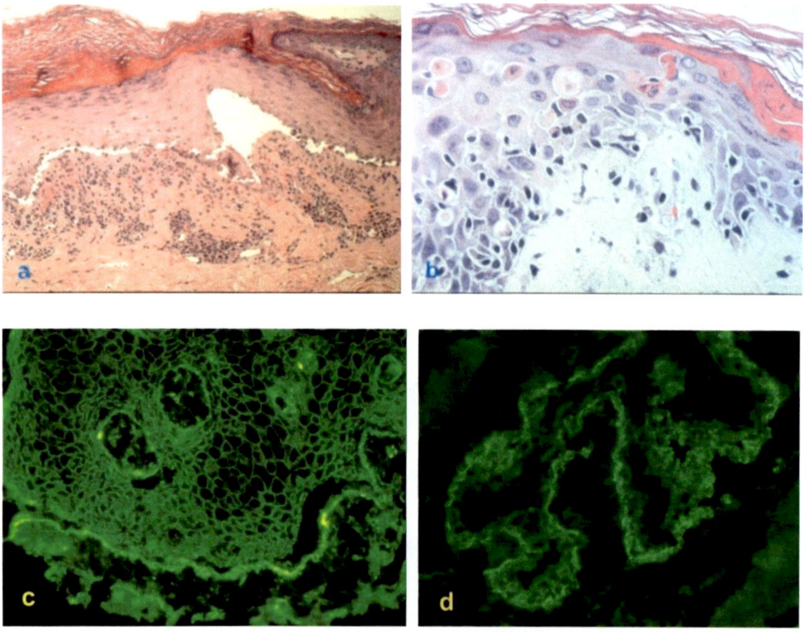

Figure 14. Histological features of paraneoplastic pemphigus delineates lichenois band-like infiltration of lymphocytes along the dermal-epidermal junction and the lower epidermal separation (a). High magnification of histology detects typical features of dyskeratotic keratinocytes (b). Immunofluorescence finding of paraneoplastic pemphigus illustrates features distinct from classic PV: DIF of a peri-lesional skin demonstrates IgG deposits both at the epidermal cell surfaces and the skin basement membrane (c). IIF on a rat bladder epithelium substrate shows that a patient with paraneoplastic pemphigus has circulating autoantibodies against the transitional epithelium (d).

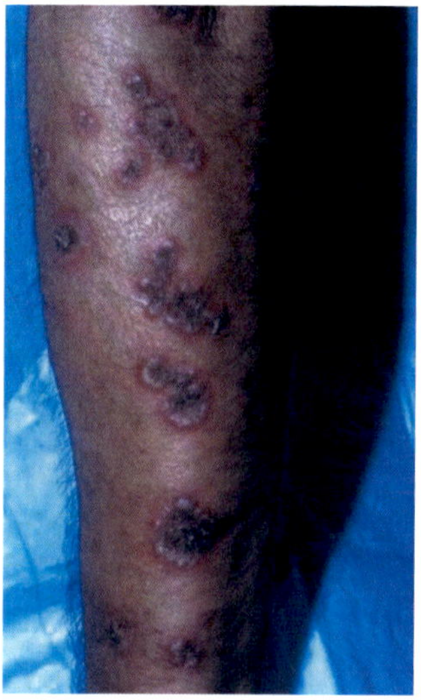

Figure 15. Clinical features of IgA pemphigus.

IV. IgA Pemphigus

As the name of the disease indicates, IgA pemphigus is mediated by the IgA class (rather than the IgG class) of autoantibodies targeting the epidermal surface protein, leading to similar, but less severe clinical manifestations. In some patients, their clinical morphology is somewhat unique and could post diagnostic challenge to the physicians, with severe oral mucosal lesions and "sunflower-like" pustular skin lesions (Tajima et al. 2010) (Figure 15). Histologically, skin biopsy from an active blister usually reveals intraepithelial blisters with neutrophilic infiltration (Wang et al. 1997, Tajima et al. 2010). By DIF, IgA was detected in the peri-lesional skin biopsy in a "chicken wiring" pattern just like that of PV (Wang et al. 1997). By IIF, IgA class circulating autoantibodies were found to bind to epithelial substrates also in a "chicken wiring" pattern (Wang et al. 1997). There appear to be two major subtypes of IgA pemphigus, with one superficial subtype where patients' IgA autoantibodies recognized an epidermal target antigen called desmocollin 1 (Tajima et al. 2010). In the other deeper subtypes, IgA class autoantibodies targeting Dsg 3 have been identified in patients (Wang et al. 1997, Robinson et al. 1999, Hashimoto et al. 2001, Tajima et al. 2010). Thus, by some measures, IgA pemphigus can be considered as a PV variant. Like other neutrophil-rich dermatoses, IgA pemphigus generally responded well to sulfur-type medication such as dapsone.

Chapter 6

Diagnostic Methodology

I. Clinical:

PV patients presented to physicians either have oral mucosal lesions or lesions of both oral mucosa and skin. Patients presented with only skin lesions are not likely to have PV. Besides oral mucosa, other mucosal areas may also be affected, such as ocular, nasal, esophageal, laryngeal, genital, and anal mucosae. Scalp and periungual areas can be involved and alopecia and severe hemorrhagic paronychia are observed in some patients. The lesions usually consist of both intact blisters and erosions, with more lesions being erosions since the blisters are easily broken, leaving behind numerous areas of small or large erosions. Blisters, if present, have a tendency to be flaccid rather than tense. If blisters are present, positive Nikolskiy's sign and Asboe-Hansen sign can be demonstrated by gently pressing with a finger at the lateral side or the top of a blister and observing the blister extension on the opposite side or the periphery of the blister, respectively. The presence of positive signs will provide additional clinical support for the diagnosis of PV. It will also be important to inquire with patients specifically about symptoms of eye irritation, dysphagia, epistaxis, hoarseness, dysuria, and pain on defecation, which will uncover potential involvement of conjunctivae, esophagus, nasal mucosae, larynx, genitaria and perianal areas.

II. Histopathology:

Skin biopsy can be obtained on an intact small blister for its entirety or on the edge of a large blister (containing both lesional and peri-lesional components). The biopsy specimen should be placed in formalin solution and processed by regular histology and stained with hematoxylin and eosin. A typical PV lesion examined under light microscope would reveal evidence of intra-epidermal blister with acantholysis, a term referred to as cell-cell separation. The blister most commonly occurs at the suprabasilar level, about one cell layer above the skin basement membrane, leaving one layer of epidermal cells attached to the skin basement membrane and an appearance of "tombstoning" (Figure 1). The reason for the last layer of epidermal cells attached is that these cells have other adhesion mechanisms to the basement membrane below, thus protecting them from being completely detached. Some inflammatory cells could be observed as well.

III. Immunofluorescence Microscopy:

A peri-lesional skin biopsy specimen can be obtained for the direct method of immunofluorescence microscopy. The biopsy specimen should be placed in normal saline in 4 C (or Michele medium in room temperature) and processed for embedding in OCT (optimal cutting temperature) compound and cryo-sectioning (frozen section). The skin sections prepared will be labeled with fluorescence-tagged antibodies against human IgG, IgM, IgA, C3, and fibrinogen. The immuno-labeled skin sections will then be examined under fluorescence microscope with epi-illumination to detect epithelial cell surface-bound IgG, or other immune components. The typical PV findings will be the presence of "chicken wiring" epithelial fluorescence pattern of IgG (and C3 as well in some cases) (Figure 2). This will confirm the diagnosis of pemphigus, but will not necessarily confirm the diagnosis of PV, as other forms of pemphigus such as PF will present the same finding. Additional tests by indirect immunofluorescence microscopy, using a patient's serum incubating with a normal epithelial substrate (commonly used monkey esophagus), followed by incubation with fluorescence-tagged antibody to human IgG and then by fluorescence microscopic examination with epi-illumination will show the same "chicken wiring" fluorescence pattern as the direct method if circulating autoantibodies are present in the patient (Figure 3).

IV. ELISA

Since ELISA is now commonly available and the cost is rather inexpensive, it has become a preferred method for confirming a diagnosis of PV, since it detects patient's circulating autoantibodies that are specific for the target antigens, Dsg 1 and Dsg 3, in the skin, in addition to being quantitative in measuring the titer of autoantibodies against specific target PV antigens.

Besides its usefulness for the initial diagnosis of PV, ELISA is also useful for management of the disease. Before a major reduction of medication during the treatment, physicians could use the data obtained from ELISA to determine the relative activities of the autoimmunity of the patients, compared to the data obtained when treatment was first initiated. A substantial reduction of ELISA-detected autoantibody titer, especially the Dsg 1 autoantibodies, provides a reasonable indicator of immunology remission, helpful for disease management (Bracke et al. 2013; Daneshpazhooh et al. 2014; Patsatsi et al. 2014; Rahbar et al. 2014; Weiss et al. 2015). Some investigators stated that initial Dsg 3 autoantibody titers are a good prognostic factor for PV (Saha et al. 2014).

Chapter 7

Therapeutic Strategies

Before we discuss the therapeutic strategies, it is appropriate to have a comprehensive overview of the specific target for each medication, with respect to the pathophysiology. Figure 16 illustrates in a schematic diagram where in the pathophysiology of PV each medication's action is targeting.

Despite many years of research into the treatment of PV, there is still no world-wide consensus on the optimal therapeutic approach, thus leaving a persistently wide variation in treatment practice (Sinha et al. 2015, McMillan et al. 2015). A systemic review according to the Cochrane Collaboration method from 2003 to 2013, based on 14 randomized/controlled clinical trials and 110 observational studies, revealed high heterogeneity in outcome measures and substantial risk of bias. This study found that 96.8% of the included studies used corticosteroids, that AZA and MMF were the most commonly cited, that there is an increasing number of studies related to biologics, and that there is insufficient quality research for optimal treatment (McMillan et al. 2015). Another systemic review and meta-analysis of randomized controlled trials compared the efficacy and safety of oral corticosteroids treatment for pemphigus, with or without adjuvants (AZA, MMF, CYC, CSP, IVIg, plasma exchange and IFX). Based on data from 10 trials consisting of 559 participants, this review found that although collectively adjuvants reduced the relapse risk by 29%, they were not beneficial for achieving remission (Atzmony et al. 2015). With respect to steroid-sparing effect, a survey gathering data from 20 studies totaling 826 participants based on Pubmed, LILACS (up to July 2014), the Cochrane Central Register of Controlled Trial (CENTRAL, issue 5 of 12, May 2014), and the ClinicalTrials.gov registry, determined that AZA had a steroid-sparing effect and did not increase remission rate. It also found that MMF induced sustained remission faster and delayed time to relapse, but did not have steroid-sparing effect, and that CYC had a steroid-sparing effect but did not affect the remission rate (Atzmony et al. 2014). Thus multicenter randomized controlled trials with uniform outcome measures are needed in the future (Atzmony et al. 2014, 2015, McMillan et al. 2015, Sinha et al. 2015).

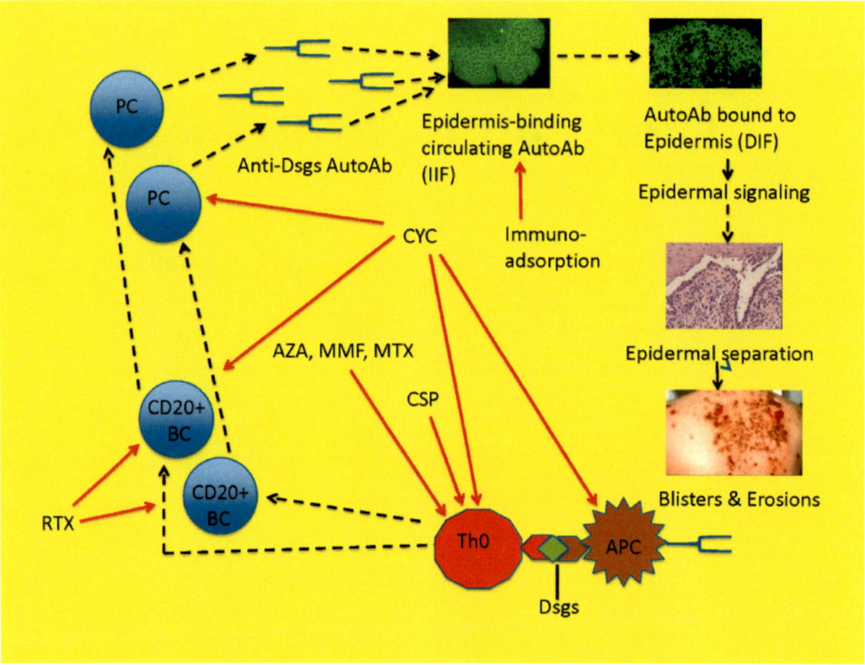

Figure 16. Schematic diagram of targeting locations of medications in reference to PV pathophysiology as depicted in Figure 5. APC, antigen presenting cells; Dsgs, desmogleins; Th0, helper T cells; BC, B cells; PC, plasma cells; AutoAb, autoantibodies; RTX, rituximab; AZA, azathioprine; MMF, mycophenolate mofetil; MTX, methotrexate; CSP, cyclosporine; CYC, Cyclophosphamide. Black dash arrows indicate the direction of immunological progression. Red solid arrows denote inhibitory actions of the medications or therapeutic method. The mechanism of disease inhibition by IVIg is not clearly defined at the present time. The disease inhibition by systemic corticosteroid may involve multiple points of this disease process.

In the absence of a consensus guideline to provide an optimal approach to treatment of PV, the following recommendations are based in part on the current literature data and the author's personal experience:

I. Localized limited oral lesion:

As mentioned in the previous section regarding clinical manifestation, some patients may present a slowly progressing oral lesion for months or even years before breaking out into generalized skin lesion. For patients initially presented with these localized, limited oral lesions, there is a dilemma as to what will be the best approach. The physician could choose a very conservative approach to utilize medications just sufficient enough to control the limited oral involvements. Alternatively, the physician could prescribe an aggressive therapeutic regimen. The real question here is whether an assertive treatment at this clinical phase of limited oral lesion suppresses the autoimmune progression, thus preventing the onset of generalized mucocutaneous disease in the future. As of today, there is no study to provide the answer to this question. Therefore, studies to this effect would be very helpful for physicians to derive an optimal treatment plan for this group of patients.

Conservative Approach

This approach aims to control the limited oral disease while minimizing side effects associated with treatments. Thus, the strategy will be to use the minimum amount of medication necessary to manage the disease. The initial treatment regimen may consist of triple medications including low dose of prednisone (30 mg daily), MMF (500-1,000 mg daily) or AZA (50-75 mg daily), and an anti-inflammatory medication (doxycycline 100 mg twice daily or dapsone 100 mg daily). It is important to initiate both the systemic corticosteroid and immunosuppressives at the very beginning so that the purpose of steroid-sparing effect can be maximized. Topical corticosteroid of mid- to high-potency can also be used as adjunct anti-inflammatory. Anti-yeast medication may also be needed to prevent oral candida infection. Topically applied cyclosporine may also be considered (Gooptu and Staughton 1998).

Assertive Approach

This approach aims not only to achieve a rapid clinical response, but also to "prevent" the possible "epitope spreading" that could lead to generalized mucocutaneous disease in the future. The initial treatment regimen may consist of triple medications including a high dose of prednisone 100 mg, MMF (1.5 g daily) or AZA (100-150 mg daily) or CYC (100 mg daily or IV pulse), and an anti-inflammatory medication (doxycycline 100 mg twice daily or dapsone 100 mg daily). Topical corticosteroid of high potency can also be used as an adjunct anti-inflammatory. Anti-yeast medication may also be needed to prevent oral candida infection.

II. Severe oral lesion:

Severe oral lesions presented in affected PV patients require a rapid action of aggressive regimen. Severe oral lesions are extremely troubling to the patients, as they are unable to properly consume food and liquid due to severe oral pain. In addition, such ingestion difficulty will inevitably result in malnutrition secondary to reduction of food consumption, affecting the general health of the patients, thereby further reducing their ability to heal. Moreover, the erosions within the oral cavity will open the door for opportunistic infection by bacteria, fungus, and other pathogens.

Therefore, the treatment regimen suggested for assertive treatment of limited oral lesion (section above) could be appropriately applied for severe oral lesion. Topical corticosteroid of high potency can also be used as adjunct anti-inflammatory. Anti-yeast medication may also be needed to prevent oral candida infection. Appropriate pain medication may also be needed to control severe symptoms of oral lesions.

III. Generalized mucocutaneous lesion:

By the time generalized skin lesions surface, it is likely that the patients already had oral mucosa lesions as well. Treatment for this group of patients naturally requires a rapid action of aggressive regimen. There is no time for medication timidity. Rapid control of skin inflammation, thereby reducing new blister formation, should be a treatment priority. Based on our knowledge that autoantibody titer correlates with disease severity, removing the circulating autoantibody should also be our treatment priority.

Thus, the strategic priorities for patients with generalized mucocutaneous manifestations are two-fold: first to quickly control the inflammation, and second to rapidly reduce the circulating autoantibody titers. To achieve the first aim, systemic corticosteroid should be initiated as soon as possible, perhaps in the dose of 1.0 to 1.5 mg/kg body weight. To accomplish the second goal, physicians have the option of applying immunosuppressives or immunoadsorption. Immunoadsorption would be a speedier way to remove the existing pathogenic IgG from circulation. On the other hand, immunosuppressives take several weeks to observe clinical effects. To prevent the production of future autoantibodies, the physicians can use either immunosuppressives or rituximab. If immunosuppressives are preferred, physicians could use MMF (1.5-2.5 g daily), AZA (100-150 mg daily) or CYC (100 mg daily or IV pulse). In addition, an anti-inflammatory medication (doxycycline 100 mg twice daily or dapsone 100 mg daily) could be added. Topical corticosteroid of high potency can also be used as adjunct anti-inflammatory. Anti-yeast medication may also be needed to prevent oral candida infection.

IV. Biologics as a first line of treatment.

The first major study investigating the use of combined RTX and IVIg for the treatment of PV was reported in 2006 (Ahmed et al. 2006). The protocol consists of three intense weekly treatments of RTX at a dose of 375 mg per m^2 body surface area, followed by a dose of IVIg at the 4th week at a dose of 2 g per kg body weight. This treatment should last for the first two months, followed by the next four months of maintenance treatment consisting of one monthly RTX and one monthly IVIg at the same doses. When using this protocol, the investigators reported a very good patient response (Ahmed et al. 2006). This study, however, treated PV patients after they failed to respond to conventional treatments. Subsequently, other protocols of RTX therapy have been studied. While some studies achieved very good clinical responses with RTX alone, other physicians emphasized that the inclusion of IVIg in the RTX regimens makes sense. The logic lies in the fact that IVIg antibodies from normal individuals who likely have received multiple vaccinations and developed immunity to a variety of common pathogens, could replace to some extent the immune defense needed for the PV patients who received anti-CD20 to deplete their B-lymphocytes and thus their antibody defense to common pathogens (Ahmed et al. 2006, Peterson and Chan 2009).

Most recently, first-line treatment of PV with a combination of RTX and high-potency topical corticosteroids has been advocated (Ingen-Housz-Oro, et al. 2015). This study included five female patients in their 50s, 60s, and 70s, who had contraindications to systemic corticosteroid treatment. These PV patients were given RTX and topical steroid resulting in favorable responses for all patients, with a mean time of clearing lesions on skin and mucosae in 15 weeks. Furthermore, two patients had no relapse at following time of 42 and 48 months. Moreover, no severe adverse effects were noted.

Thus, RTX can be used as a first-line treatment instead of using it as a last resort after failing the conventional treatments of systemic corticosteroid and immunosuppressives. This will be particularly useful for patients to whom the use of systemic corticosteroid or immunosuppressive will be contraindicated. The author still believes that these patients who received RTX treatment would also benefit from receiving periodic treatment of IVIg, not only as an adjunct treatment for PV, but also as a preventative measure to supplement a patient's antibody-mediated immune function during a time when the patient's antibody defense is at its minimum. A monthly dose of IVIg (2 g/kg) for six months after receiving RTX would be a reasonable consideration.

V. Monitoring treatment side effects on the immune system:

A nationwide population-based study in Taiwan revealed that the overall mortality rate of PV patients is more than twice that of the general population. One of the major causes of mortality in this study is infection/septicemia (Huang et al. 2012). A UK population-based survey also reported an overall mortality rate of PV patients being more than three times that of the general population (Langan et al. 2008). Medication side effects may in part contribute to this increased mortality rate.

With PV patients on systemic corticosteroid, immunosuppressives, or biologics treatments, the functions of their immune system are partially reduced and they are vulnerable to developing more serious infection and even neoplasm. It is therefore very important to monitor carefully any early signs of such adverse medication effects and to correct these side effects in a timely fashion before it is too late.

A. Monitor side effects by symptoms:

During patients' follow-up visits, the managing physicians can inquire about the following symptoms relevant to side effects of medical regimen, with regard to bone marrow over suppression:

1. Frequent infection
2. Delayed recovery after an infection
3. Shortness of breath on minimum exertion
4. Easy to feel tired
5. Bloody diarrhea, black or tarry stool
6. General malaise
7. Easy bruising

B. Monitor side effects by laboratory tests:

Patients on immunosuppressives treatment should have periodic tests for complete blood count with differential analysis and absolute count of various white cells. One of the early manifestations of over suppression will be a substantial drop of absolute lymphocyte count. Since the therapeutic purpose of immunosuppressives (particularly AZA and MMF) is to reduce the lymphocyte count in controlling the disease, the question is what level of lymphocyte suppression will be appropriate for controlling the disease and yet still reserve sufficient immune defense for the patients. Some physicians choose a value of absolute lymphocyte count at its 50% of lower normal range as a "line on the sand," below which bone marrow will be considered over suppression that requires a reduction of medication. Screening complete blood count will detect the unlikely scenario of pancytopenia.

VI. Monitor treatment side effects on metabolic system:

The importance of monitoring metabolic side effects of medication is mainly for patients receiving systemic corticosteroid treatment.

A. Monitor side effects by symptoms:
1. Symptoms of psychosis
2. Sleep trouble
3. Significant weight gain
4. Polyuria and polydipsia

5. Delayed wound healing
6. Vision impairment

B. Monitor side effects by laboratory methods:
1. Periodic fasting blood sugar
2. Periodic urine analysis
3. Periodic bone density scan

VII. Monitor medication-specific side effects:

A. AZA: Since AZA and other immunosuppressives can cause liver toxicity, it will be prudent to monitor blood liver enzymes regularly for patients on these immunosuppressives. Patients with acute or chronic liver disease should not be treated with AZA. In addition, thiopurine S-methyltransferase activity (TPMT) should be monitored for all Caucasian and African patients treated with AZA, although study did not indicate its usefulness (Firooz et al. 2008, el-Azhary et al. 2009, Meyer and Beissert 2012). Patients of Japanese origin should be screened for inosine triphosphate pyrophosphohydrolase (ITPA) activity instead (Meyer and Beissert 2012). Since TPMT functions to clear azathioprine from the body system, a low TPMT level posts a higher chance of toxicity, necessitating a lower dose of medication. Pancreatitis can also be a side effect of AZA.
B. CYC: One particular problem for patients receiving CYC treatment is the potential side effect of hemorrhagic cystitis. Thus, regularly monitoring this side effect by urine analysis will be important. Patients with acute or chronic urinary bladder disease should not be treated with CYC.
C. CSP: The known renal toxicity of CSP requires close monitoring of this organ-specific side effect. Patients with acute or chronic renal disease should not be treated with CSP.
D. MTX: Since MTX has well-recognized liver toxicity, regular monitoring of patients' blood liver enzymes needs to be performed. Patients with acute or chronic liver disease should not be treated with MTX. Furthermore, patients being treated with MTX should receive a daily dose of folate on days that MTX is not taken. Periodic liver biopsy may be required for long-term MTX usage.

E. IVIg: Patients with cardiovascular diseases, immobility, hypertension, and thrombotic events probably should not be treated with IVIg.
F. Dapsone: Patients with sulfur allergy is a relative contraindication for taking dapsone. G6PD level should be checked for all patients receiving dapsone.

References

Aboobaker J, Morar N, Ramdial PK, Hammond MG. Pemphigus in South Africa. *Int. J. Dermatol.* 2001; 40:115-9.

Ahmed AR, Hombal S. Use of cyclophosphamide in azathioprine failures in pemphigus. *J. Am. Acad. Dermatol.* 1987; 17:437-42.

Ahmed AR, Spigelman Z, Cavacini LA, Posner MR. Treatment of pemphigus vulgaris with rituximab and intravenous immune globulin. *New Engl. J. Med.* 2006; 355:1772-9.

Ahmed AR, Shetty S. A comprehensive analysis of treatment outcomes in patients with pemphigus vulgaris treated with rituximab. *Autoimmun. Rev.* 2015; 14:323-31.

Aksoy S, Arslan C, Harputluoglu H, Dizdar O, Altundag K. Malignancies after rituximab treatment: just coincidence or more? *J. BUON* 2011; 16:112-5.

Al-Harbi TM, Al-Muammar SA, Ellis RJ. Brain abscess following rituximab infusion in a patient with pemphigus vulgaris. *Am. J. Case Resp.* 2015; 16:65-8.

Alijotas J, Pedragosa R, Bosch J, Vilardell M. Prolonged remission after cyclosporine therapy in pemphigus vulgaris: report of two young siblings. *J. Am. Acad. Dermatol.* 1990; 23:701-3.

Amagai M, Klaus-Kovtun V, Stanley JR. Autoantibodies against a novel epithelial cadherin in pemphigus vulgaris, a disease of cell adhesion. *Cell* 1991; 67:869-77.

Amagai M, Nishikawa T, Nousari HC, Anhalt GJ, Hashimoto T. Antibodies against desmoglein 3 (pemphigus vulgaris antigen) are present in sera from patients with paraneoplastic pemphigus and cause acantholysis in vivo in neonatal mice. *J. Clin. Invest.* 1998; 102:775-82.

Amagai M, Tsunoda K, Suzuki H, Nishifuji K, Koyasu S, Nishikawa T. Use of autoantigen-knockout mice in developing an active autoimmune disease model for pemphigus. *J. Clin. Invest.* 2000; 105:625-31.

Amagai M. Pemphigus vulgaris and its active disease mouse model. *Curr. Dir. Autoimmun.* 2008; 10:167-81.

Amber KT, Staropoli P, Shiman MI, Elgart GW, Hertl M. Autoreactive T cells in the immune pathogenesis of pemphigus vulgaris. *Exp. Dermatol.* 2013; 22:699-704.

Amber KT, Hertl M. An assessment of treatment history and its association with clinical outcomes and relapse in 155 pemphigus patients with response to a single cycle or rituximab. *J. Eur. Acad. Dermatol. Venereol.* 2015; 29:777-82.

Amichai B, Grunwald MH, Gasper N, Finkelstein E, Halevy S. A case of pemphigus vulgaris with esophageal involvement. *J. Dermatol.* 1996; 23:214-5.

Anhalt GJ, Labib RS, Voorhees JJ, Beals TF, Diaz LA. Induction of pemphigus in neonatal mice by passive transfer from patients with the disease. *N. Engl. J. Med.* 1982; 306:1189-96.

Anhalt GJ, Kim SC, Stanley JR, et al. Paraneoplastic pemphigus. An autoimmune mucocutaneous disease associated with neoplasm. *N. Engl. J. Med.* 1990; 323:1729-35.

Anhalt GJ. Paraneoplastic pemphigus. Adv Dermatol 1997; 12:77-96.

Anhalt GJ. Paraneoplastic pemphigus. *J. Invest. Dermatol. Symp. Proc.* 2004; 9:29-33.

Asarch A, Swick BL, Fairley JA. Cryptic esophageal pemphigus vulgaris despite apparent clinical remission. *J. Am. Acad. Dermatol.* 2012; 67:e213-4. Doi:10.1016/j.jaad.2012.03.003.

Asboe-Hansen G. Blister-spreading induced by finger-pressure, a diagnostic sign in pemphigus. *J. Invest. Dermatol.* 1960; 34:5-9.

Asboe-Hansen G. Blister spreading, a diagnostic test in pemphigus. Loss of epidermal and dermoepidermal cohesion. *Arch. Dermatol. Res.* 1988; 280:suppl S66-7.

Atzmony L, Hodak E, Gdalevich M, Rosenbaum O, Mimouni D. Treatment of pemphigus vulgaris and pemphigus foliaceus: a systematic review and meta-analysis. *Am. J. Clin. Dermatol.* 2014; 15:503-15.

Atzmony L, Hodak E, Leshem YA, et al. The role of adjuvant therapy in pemphigus: A systemic review and meta-analysis. *J. Am. Acad. Dermatol.* 2015; 73:264-71.

Baican A, Baican C, Chiriac G, et al. Pemphigus vulgaris is the most common autoimmune bullous disease in Northwestern Romania. *Int. J. Dermatol.* 2010; 49:768-74.

Balighi K, Daneshpazhooh M, Khezri S, Mahdavi-nia M, Hajiseyed-javadi M, Chams-Davatchi C. Adjuvant rituximab in the treatment of pemphigus vulgaris: a phase II clinical trial. *Int. J. Dermatol.* 2013; 52:862-7.

Barnadas M, Roe E, Brunet S, et al. Therapy of paraneoplastic pemphigus with rituximab: a case report and review of literature. *J. Eur. Acad. Dermatol. Venereol.* 2006; 20:69-74.

Baroni A, Russo T, Faccenda F, Piccolo V. Amoxicillin/clavulanic acid-induced pemphigus vulgaris: case report. *Acta Dermatovenerol. Croat* 2012; 20:108-11.

Barthelemy H, Frappaz A, Cambazard F, et al. Treatment of nine cases of pemphigus vulgaris with cyclosporine. *J. Am. Acad. Dermatol.* 1988; 18:1262-6.

Baum S, Greenberger S, Samuelov L, et al. Methotrexate is an effective and safe adjuvant therapy for pemphigus vulgaris. *Eur. J. Dermatol.* 2012; 22:83-7.

Beissert S, Werfel T, Frieling U, et al. A comparison of oral methylprednisolone plus azathioprine or mycophenolate mofetil for the treatment of pemphigus. *Arch. Dermatol.* 2006; 142:1447-54.

Beissert S, Werfel T, Frieling U. et al. A comparison of oral methylprednisolone plus azathioprine or mycophenolate mofetil for the treatment of bullous pemphigoid. *Arch. Dermatol.* 2007; 143:1536-42.

Beissert S, Mimouni D, Kanwar AJ, Solomons N, Kalia V, Anhalt GJ. Treating pemphigus vulgaris with prednisone and mycophenolate mofetil: a multicenter, randomized, placebo-controlled trial. *J. Invest. Dermatol.* 2010; 130:2041-8.

Bektas M, Jolly P, Rubenstein DS. Apoptotic pathways in pemphigus. *Dermatol. Res. Pract.* 2010; 2010:456841. Doi:10.1155/2010/456841.

Bektas M, Jolly PS, Berkowitz P, Amagai M, Rubenstein DS. A pathophysiologic role for epidermal growth factor receptor in pemphigus acantholysis. *J. Biol. Chem.* 2013; 288:9447-56.

Ben Salem C, Ben Salah L, Belajouza C, Bouraoui K. Azathioprine-induced severe cholestatic hepatitis in patient carrying TPMT*3C polymorphism. *Pharm. World Sci.* 2010; 32:701-3.

Berkowitz P, Hu P, Liu Z, et al. Desmosome signaling. Inhibition of p38MAPK prevents pemphigus vulgaris IgG-induced cytoskeleton reorganization. *J. Biol. Chem.* 2005; 280:23778-84.

Berkowitz P, Hu P, Warren S, Liu Z, Diaz LA, Rubenstein DS. P38MAPK inhibition prevents disease in pemphigus vulgaris mice. *Proc. Natl. Acad. Sci. USA* 2006; 103:12855-60.

Berkowitz P, Diaz LA, Hall RP, Rubenstein DS. Induction of p38MAPK and HSP27 phosphorylation in pemphigus patient skin. *J. Invest. Dermatol.* 2008; 128:738-40.

Beutner EH, Jordon RE. Demonstration of skin antibodies in sera of pemphigus vulgaris patients by indirect immunofluorescent staining. *Proc. Soc. Exp. Biol. Med.* 1964; 117:505-10.

Beutner EH, Lever WF, Witebskyu E, Jordon R, Chertock B. Autoantibodies in pemphigus vulgaris: Response to an intercellular substance of epidermis. *JAMA* 1965; 24:682-8.

Bewley AP, Keefe M. Successful treatment of pemphigus vulgaris by pulsed intravenous immunoglobulin therapy. *Br. J. Dermatol.* 1996; 135:128-9.

Bhanusali DG, Sachdev A, Rahmanian A, et al. HLA-E*0103X is associated with susceptibility to pemphigus vulgaris. *Exp. Dermatol.* 2013; 22:108-12.

Bowen GM, Peters NT, Fivenson DP, et al. Lichenoid dermatitis in paraneoplastic pemphigus: a pathogenic trigger of epitope spreading? *Arch. Dermatol.* 2000; 136:652-6.

Bozdaq K, Bilqin I. Epidemiology of pemphigus in the western region of Turkey: retrospective analysis of 87 patients. *Cutan Ocul. Toxicol* 2012; 31:280-5.

Bracke S, Speekaert R, Van Geel N, De Bacquer D, Lambert J. Evaluation of commercially available ELISA assays as a tool for monitoring and managing pemphigus patients: a prospective study. *Eur. J. Dermatol.* 2013; 23:33-9.

Brenner S, Bialy-Golan A, Anhalt GJ. Recognition of pemphigus antigens in drug-induced pemphigus vulgaris and pemphigus foliaceus. *J. Am. Acad. Dermatol.* 1997; 36:919-23.

Bystryn JC, Jiao D. IVIg selectively and rapidly decreases circulating pathogenic autoantibodies in pemphigus vulgaris. *Autoimmunity* 2006; 39:601-7.

Caldarola G, Carbone A, De Simone C, Pellicano R. Development of pemphigus vulgaris in a patient with psoriasis treated with cyclosporine. *J. Am. Acad. Dermatol.* 2010; 63:356-7.

Chaidemenos G, Apalla Z, Koussidou T, Papagarifallou I, Ioannides D. High dose oral prednisone vs. prednisone plus azathioprine for the treatment of oral pemphigus: a retrospective, bi-centre, comparative study. *J. Eur. Acad. Dermatol. Venereol.* 2011; 25:106-10.

Chams-Davatchi C, Esmaili N, Daneshapazhooh, M, et al. Randomized controlled open-label trial of four treatment regimens for pemphigus vulgaris. *J. Am. Acad. Dermatol.* 2007; 57:622-8.

Chams-Davatchi C, Mortazavizadeh A, Daneshpazhooh M, et al. Randomized double blind trial of prednisone and azathioprine, vs. prednisone and placebo, in the treatment of pemphigus vulgaris. *J. Eur. Acad. Dermatol. Venereol.* 2013; 27:1285-92.

Chan LS, Vanderlugt C, Hashimoto T, et al. Epitope spreading: lessons from autoimmune skin diseases. *J. Invest. Dermatol.* 1998; 110:103-9.

Chan LS. Epitope spreading in paraneoplastic pemphigus: autoimmune induction in antibody-mediated blistering skin diseases. *Arch. Dermatol.*. 2000;136:663-4.

Chan LS and Pappo EL. Malignancy risk is not demonstrated in patients with immunobullous diseases receiving mycophenolate mofetil. *J. Invest. Dermatol.* 2013; 133:S94 (Abstract No. 550).

Chernyavsky A, Chen Y, Wang PH, Grando SA. Pemphigus vulgaris antibodies target the mitochondrial nicotinic acetylcholine receptors that protect keratinocytes from apoptolysis. *Int. Immunopharmacol.* 2015; May 18.

Cho YT, Lee FY, Chu CY, Wang LF. First-line combination therapy with rituximab and corticosteroids is effective and safe for pemphigus. *Acta Derm. Venereol.* 2014; 94:472-3.

Chyama M, Amagai M, Tsunoda K, Ota T, Koyasu S, Hata J, Umezawa A, Nishikawa T. Immunologic and histopathologic characterization of an active disease model for pemphigus vulgaris. *J. Invest. Dermatol.* 2002; 118:199-204.

Civatte A. Diagnostic histopathologique de la dermatite polymorphe douloureuse ou maladie de Duhring-Brocq. *Ann. Dermatol. Syph.* 1943; 3:1-30.

Clifford KS, Demierre MF. Progression of classic Kaposi's sarcoma with rituximab. *J. Am. Acad. Dermatol.* 2005; 53:155-7.

Colliou N, Picard D, Caillot F, et al. Long-term remissions of severe pemphigus after rituximab therapy are associated with prolonged failure of desmoglein B cell response. *Sci. Transl. Med.* 2013; 5:175ra30.

Cozzani E[1], Christana K, Mastrogiacomo A, et al. Pemphigus vegetans Neumann type with anti-desmoglein and anti-periplakin autoantibodies. *Eur. J. Dermatol.* 2007; 17:530-3.

Culton DA, McCray SK, Park M, et al. Mucosal pemphigus vulgaris anti-Dsg3 IgG is pathogenic to oral mucosa of humanized Dsg3 mice. *J. Invest. Dermatol.* 2015; 135:1590-7.

Cummins DL, Mimouni D, Anhalt GJ, Nousari CH. Oral cyclophosphamide for treatment of pemphigus vulgaris and foliaceus. *J. Am. Acad. Dermatol.* 2003; 49:276-80.

Czernik A, Camilleri M, Pittelkow MR, Grando SA. Paraneoplastic autoimmune multiorgan syndrome: 20 years later, *Int. J. Dermatol.* 2011; 50:905-14.

Daneshpazhooh M, Moeineddin F, Kiani A, et al. Fatal paraneoplastic pemphigus after removal of Cattleman's disease in a child. *Pediatr Dermatol.* 2012; 29:656-7.

Daneshpazhooh M, Kamyab K, Kalantari MS, et al. Comparison of desmoglein 1 and 3 enzyme-linked immunosorbent assay and direct immunofluorescence for evaluation of immunological remission in pemphigus vulgaris. *Clin. Exp. Dermatol.* 2014; 39:41-7.

Ding X, Aoki V, Mascaro JM, Lopez-Swiderski A, Diaz LA, Fairley JA. Mucosal and mucocutaneous (generalized) pemphigus vulgaris show distinct autoantibody profiles. *J. Invest. Dermatol.* 1997; 109:592-6.

Duhring A. Dermatitis herpetiformis (reprinted from JAMA 1884; 3:225-9). *JAMA* 1983; 250:212-6.

Durdu M, Baba M, Seckin D. The value of Tzanck smear test in diagnosis of erosive, vesicular, bullous, and pustular skin lesions. *J. Am. Acad. Dermatol.* 2008; 59:958-64.

El-Azhary RA, Farmer SA, Drage LA, et al. Thioguanine nucleotides and thiopurine methyltransferase in immunobullous diseases: optimal levels as adjunctive tools for azathioprine monitoring. *Arch. Dermatol.* 2009; 145:644-52.

Ellebrecht CT, Choi EJ, Allman DM, et al. Subcutaneous veltuzumab, a humanized anti-CD20 antibody, in the treatment of refractory pemphigus vulgris. *JAMA Dermatol.* 2014; 150:1331-5.

Eming R, Hennerici T, Backlund J. et al. Pathogenic IgG antibodies against desmoglein 3 in pemphigus vulgaris are regulated by HLA-DRB1*04:02-restricted T cells. *J. Immunol.* 2014; 193:4391-9.

FDA: What are "biologics" questions and answers. (www.fda.gov) accessed October 3, 2015.

Fellner MJ, Katz JM, McCable JB. Successful use of cyclophosphamide and prednisone for initial treatment of pemphigus vulgaris. *Arch. Dermatol.* 1978; 114:889-94.

Feng S, Zhou W, Zhang J, Jin P. Analysis of 6 cases of drug-induced pemphigus. *Eur. J. Dermatol.* 2011; 21:696-9.

Fernandez S, Espana A, Navedo M, Barona L. Study of oral, ear, nose and throat involvement in pemphigus vulgaris by endoscopic examination. *Br. J. Dermatol.* 2012; 167:1011-6.

Firooz A, Ghandi N, Hallaji Z, Chams-Davatchi C, Valikhani M, Karbakhsh Davari M. Role of thiopurine methyltransferase activity in the safety and efficacy of azathioprine in the treatment of pemphigus vulgaris. *Arch. Dermatol.* 2008; 144:1143-7.

Frew JW, Murrell DF. Paraneoplastic pemphigus (paraneoplastic autoimmune multiorgan syndrome): clinical presentations and pathogenesis. *Dermatol. Clin.* 2011; 29:419-25.

Fullerton SH, Woodley DT, Smoller BR, Anhalt GJ. Paraneoplastic pemphigus with autoantibody deposition in bronchial epithelium after autologous bone marrow transplantation. *JAMA* 1992; 267:1500-2.

Gammon WR, Briggaman RA, Wheeler CE, Jr. Epidermolysis bullosa acquisita presenting as an inflammatory bullous disease. *J. Am. Acad. Dermatol.* 1982; 7:382-7.

Gholizadeh N, Taghavi Zenouz A, Eslami H. Pemphigus vulgaris associated with rheumatoid arthritis in a patient not taking penicillamine. *J. Dent. Res. Dent. Clin. Dent. Prospects* 2102; 6:33-5.

Gooptu C, Staughton RC. Use of topical cyclosporine in oral pemphigus. *J. Am. Acad. Dermatol.* 1998; 38:860-1.

Grando SA, Grando AA, Glukhensky BT, Doguzov V, Nguyen VT, Holubar K. History and clinical significance of mechanical symptoms in blistering dermatoses: a reappraisal. *J. Am. Acad. Dermatol.* 2003; 48:86-92.

Grando SA, Bystryn JC, Chernyavsky AI, et al. Apoptolysis: a novel mechanism of skin blistering in pemphigus vulgaris linking the apoptotic pathways to basal dell shrinkage and suprabasal acantholysis. *Exp. Dermatol.* 2009; 18:764-70.

Grando SA, Pittelkow MR. Pseudo pemphigus phenotype in mice with inactivated desmoglein 3: Further insight to the complexity of pemphigus pathophysiology. *Am. J. Pathol.* 2015; 185:3125-7.

Gregorious S, Giatrakou S, Theodoropoulos K, et al. Pilot study of 19 patients with severe pemphigus: prophylactic treatment with rituximab does not appear to be beneficial. *Dermatology* 2014; 228:158-65.

Guilloteau K, Paris I, Pedretti N, et al. Skin inflammation induced by the synergistic action of IL-17A, IL-22, Oncostatin M, IL-1a, and TNF-a recapitulates some features of psoriasis. *J. Immunol.* 2010; 184:5263-70.

Gunther C. Laske J, Frind A, Julius U, Pfeiffer C. Successful therapy of pemphigus vulgaris with immunoadsorption using the TheraSorb adsorber. *J. Dtsch. Dermatol. Ges.* 2008; 6:661-3.

Hadayer N, Ramot Y, Maly A, Zlotogorski A. Pemphigus vulgaris with loss of hair on the scalp. *Int. J. Trichology* 2013; 5:157-8.

Hall RP, Fairley J, Woodley D, et al. A multicentre randomized trial of the treatment of patients with pemphigus vulgaris with infliximab and prednisone compared to prednisone alone. *Br. J. Dermatol.* 2015; 172:760-8.

Hashimoto K[1], Hashimoto T, Higashiyama M, Nishikawa T, Garrod DR, Yoshikawa K. Detection of anti-desmocollins I and II autoantibodies in two cases of Hallopeau type pemphigus vegetans by immunoblot analysis. *J. Dermatol. Sci* 1994;7:100-6.

Hashimoto T, Kormai A, Futei Y, Nishikawa T, Amagai M. Detection of IgA autoantibodies to desmogleins by an enzyme-linked immunosorbent assay: the presence of new minor subtypes of IgA pemphigus. *Arch. Dermatol.* 2001; 137:735-8.

Hashizume H[1], Iwatsuki K, Takigawa M. Epidermal antigens and complement-binding anti-intercellular antibodies in pemphigus vegetans, Hallopeau type. *Br. J. Dermatol.*. 1993;129:739-43.

Heelan K, Al-Mohammedi F, Smith MJ, et al. Durable remission of pemphigus with a fixed-dose rituximab protocol. *JAMA Dermatol.* 2014; 150:703-8.

Heizmann M, Itin P, Wernli M, Borradori L, Bargetzi MJ. Successful treatment of paraneoplastic pemphigus in follicular NHL with rituximab: report of a case and review of treatment for paraneoplastic pemphigus in NHL and CLL. *Am. J. Hematol.* 2001; 66:142-4.

Helou J, Allbritton J, Anhalt GJ. Accuracy of indirect immunofluorescence testing in the diagnosis of paraneoplastic pemphigus. *J. Acad. Dermatol.* 1995; 32:441-7.

Hodak E, Kremer I, David M, et al. Conjunctival involvement in pemphigus vulgaris: a clinical, histopathological and immunofluorescence study. *Br. J. Dermatol.* 1990; 123:615-20.

Hoffman MA, Qiao X, Anhalt GJ. CD8+ T lymphocytes in bronchiolitis obliterans, paraneoplastic pemphigus, and solitary Castleman's disease. *N. Engl. J. Med.* 2003; 349:407-8.

Horn TD, Anhalt GJ. Histologic features of paraneoplastic pemphigus. *Arch. Dermatol.* 1992; 128:1091-5.

Huang YH, Kuo CF, Chen YH, Yang YW. Incidence, mortality, and causes of death of patients with pemphigus in Taiwan: a nationwide population-based study. *J. Invest. Dermatol.* 2012; 132:92-7.

Ingen-Housz-Oro S, Valeyrie-Allanore L, Cosnes A, Ortonne N, Hue S, Paul M, Wolkenstein P, Chosidow O. First-line treatment of pemphigus vulgaris with a combination of rituximab and high-potency topical croticosteroids. *JAMA Dermatol.* 2015; 151:2000-3.

Ioannides D, Chrysomallis F, Bystryn JC. Ineffectiveness of cyclosporine as an adjuvant to corticosteroids in the treatment of pemphigus. *Arch. Dermatol.* 2000; 136:868-72.

Jackson GT. Dermatological Bibliography. Press of Stettimer, Lambert & Co., New York, NY 1891, p77.

Jolly PS, Berkowitz P, Bektas M, et al. p38MAPK signaling and desmoglein-3 internalization are linked events in pemphigus acantholysis. *J. Biol. Chem.* 2010; 285:8936-41.

Kalantari-Dehaghi M, Chen Y, Deng W, et al. Mechanisms of mitochondrial damage in keratinocytes by pemphigus vulgaris antibodies. *J. Biol. Chem.* 2013; 288:16916-25.

Kamphausen I, Schulze F, Schmidt E, Zillikens D, Kunz M. Treatment of severe pemphigus vulgaris of the scalp with adjuvant rituximab and immunoadsorption. *Eur. J. Dermatol.* 2012; 22:786-7.

Kanwar AJ, Kaur S, Thami GP. Long-term efficacy of dexamethasone-cyclophosphamide pulse therapy in pemphigus. *Dermatology* 2002; 204:228-31.

Kanwar AJ, Vinay K, Sawatkar GU, et al. Clinical and immunological outcomes of high-and low-dose rituximab treatments in patients with pemphigus: a randomized, comparative, observer-blinded study. *Br. J. Dermatol.* 2014; 170:1341-9.

Karpati S, Amagai M, Prussick R, Cehrs K, Stanley JR. Pemphigus vulgaris antigen, a desmoglein type of cadherin, is localized within keratinocyte desmosomes. *J. Cell Biol.* 1993; 122:409-15.

Kasperkiewicz M, Shimanovich I, Meier M, et al. Treatment of severe pemphigus with a combination of immunoadsorption, rituximab, pulsed dexamethasone and azathioprine/mycophenolate mofetil: a pilot study of 23 patients. *Br. J. Dermatol.* 2012; 166:154-60.

Khamaysi I, Eliakim R. Esophageal pemphigus vulgaris: a rare manifestation revisited. *Gastroenterol. Hepatol. (NY)* 2008; 4:71-2.

King DF, Holubar K. History of pemphigus. *Clin. Dermatol.* 1983; 1:6-12.

Kljuic A, Bazzi H, Sundberg JP, et al. Desmoglein 4 in hair follicle differentiation and epidermal adhesion: evidence from inherited hypotrichosis and acquired pemphigus vulgaris. *Cell* 2003;113:249-60.

Koch PJ, Mahoney MG, Ishikawa H, et al. Target disruption of the pemphigus vulgaris (desmoglein 3) gene in mice causes loss of keratinocyte cell adhesion with a phenotype similar to pemphigus vulgaris. *J. Cell Biol.* 1997; 137:1091-102.

Korman NJ, Eyre RW, Zone J, Stanley JR. Drug-induced pemphigus: autoantibodies directed against the pemphigus antigen complexes are present in penicillamine and captopril-induced pemphigus. *J. Invest. Dermatol.* 1991; 96:273-6.

Kulthanan K, Chularojanamontri L, Tuchinda P, Sirikudta W, Pinkaew S. Clinical features and course of pemphigus in Thai patients. *Asian Pac. J. Allergy Immunol.* 2011; 29:161-8.

Landau M, Brenner S. Histologic findings in drug-induced pemphigus. *Am. J. Dermatopathol.* 1997; 19:411-4.

Lane JE, Woody C, Davis LS, Guill MF, Jerath RS. Paraneoplastic autoimmune multiorgan syndrome (paraneoplastic pemphigus) in a child: case report and review of the literature. *Pediatrics* 2004; 114:e513-6.

Langan SM, Smeeth L, Hubbard R, Fleming KM, Smith CJ, West J. Bullous pemphigoid and pemphigus vulgaris-incidence and mortality in the UK: population based cohort study. *BMJ* 2008; July 9, 337:a180. Doi: 10.1136/bmj.a180.

Lapidoth M, David M, Ben-Amitai D, Katzenelson V, Lustig S, Sandbank M. The efficacy of combined treatment with prednisone and cyclosporine in patients with pemphigus: preliminary study. *J. Am. Acad. Dermatol.* 1994; 30:752-7.

Lee E, Lendas KA, Chow S. et al. Disease relevant HLA class II alleles isolated by genotypic, haplotypic, and sequence analysis in North American Caucasians with pemphigus vulgaris. *Hum. Immunol.* 2006; 67:125-39.

Leshem YA, David M, Hodak E, et al. A prospective study on clinical response and cell-mediated immunity of pemphigus patients treated with rituximab. *Arch. Dermatol. Res.* 2014; 306:67-74.

Lever WF. Pemphigus: a histologic study. *AMA Arch. Dermatol. Syphilol.* 1951; 64:727-53.

Lever WF. Pemphigus. *Medicine (Baltimore).* 1953; 32:1-123.

Lever WF, White H. Treatment of pemphigus with corticosteroids. Results obtained in 46 patients over a period of 11 years. *Arch. Dermatol.* 1963; 87:12-26.

Lever WF, Schaumburg-Lever G. Immunosuppressants and prednisone in pemphigus vulgaris: therapeutic results obtained in 63 patients between 1961 and 1975. *Arch. Dermatol.* 1977; 113:1236-41.

Lever WF, Schaumburg-Lever G. Treatment of pemphigus vulgaris. Results obtained in 84 patients between 1961 and 1982. *Arch. Dermatol.* 1984; 120:44-7.

Li WW, Chen XX, Yu J, Wang Y, Bu DF, Tu P. Haemolytic anemia following rituximab treatment in a patient with pemphigus vulgaris. *Br. J. Dermatol.* 2009; 161:205-6.

Lin MS, Swartz SJ, Lopez A, et al. Development and characterization of desmoglein-3 specific T cells from patients with pemphigus vulgaris. *J. Clin. Invest.* 1997; 99:31-40.

Mahmoud A, Miziara ID, Costa KC, Santi CG, Maruta CW, Aoki V. Laryngeal involvement in pemphigus vulgaris: a proposed classification. *J. Laryngol. Otol.* 2012; 126:1041-4.

Mahoney MG, Wang Z, Rothenberger K, Koch PJ, Amagai M, Stanley JR. Explanations for the clinical and microscopic localization of lesions in pemphigus foliaceus and vulgaris. *J. Clin. Invest.* 1999; 103:461-8.

Mao X, Sano Y, Park JM, Payne AS. P38 MARK activation is downstream of the loss of intercellular adhesion in pemphigus vulgaris. *J. Biol. Chem.* 2011; 286:1283-91.

Marchenko S, Chernyavsky AI, Arredondo J, Gindi V, Grando SA. Antimitochondrial autoantibodies in pemphigus vulgaris: a missing link in disease pathophysiology. *J. Biol. Chem.* 2010; 285:3695-704.

Matsuda S, Koyasu S. Mechanisms of action of cyclosporine. *Immunopharmacology* 2000; 47:119-25.

McMillan R, Taylor J, Shephard M, et al. World workshop on oral medicine VI: a systemic review of the treatment of mucocutaneous pemphigus vulgaris. *Oral. Surg. Oral. Med. Oral. Pathol. Oral. Radiol.* 2015; 120:132-42.

Meyer V, Beissert S. Azathioprine in the treatment of autoimmune blistering diseases. *Immunol. Allergy Clin. North Am.* 2012; 32:296-307.

Mignogna MD, Fedele S, Lo Russo L, Bonadies G, Nappa S, Lo Muzio L. Acute cyclosporine nephrotoxicity in a patient with oral pemphigus vulgaris and HIV infection on antiretroviral therapy. *J. Am. Acad. Dermatol.* 2005; 53:1089-90.

Mimouni D, Anhalt GJ, Lazarova Z, et al. Paraneoplastic pemphigus in children and adolescents. *Br. J. Dermatol.* 2002; 147:725-32.

Mobini N, Padilla T Jr, Ahmed AR. Long-term remission in selected patients with pemphigus vulgaris treated with cyclosporine. *J. Am. Acad. Dermatol.* 1997; 36:264-6.

Munhoz Ede A, Cardoso CL, Barreto JA, Soares CT, Damante JH. Severe manifestation of oral pemphigus. *Am. J. Otolaryngol.* 2011; 32:338-42.

Nguyen T, Ahmed AR. Pemphigus vulgaris localized to the tongue. *J. Dermatol. Case Rep.* 2014; 8:55-7.

Nguyen VT, Ndoye A, Bassler KD, et al. Classification, clinical manifestations, and immunopathological mechanisms of the epithelial variant of paraneoplastic autoimmune multiorgan syndrome: a reappraisal of paraneoplastic pemphigus. *Arch. Dermatol.* 2001; 137:193-206.

Oettinger-Barak O, Machtei EE, Peled M, Barak S, L-Naaj IA, Laufer D. Cyclosporine A-induced gingival hyperplasia pemphigus vulgaris: literature review and report of a case. *J. Periodontol.* 2000; 71:650-6.

Ogata K, Yasuda K, Matsushita M, Kodama H. Successful treatment of adolescent pemphigus vulgaris by immunoadsorption method. *J. Dermatol.* 1999; 26:236-9.

Ohata Y, Komiya H, Kawahara Y, Watanabe K, Nishikawa T, Hashimoto T. A case of Neumann type pemphigus vegetans showing reactivity with the 130 kD pemphigus vulgaris antigen. *Acta Derm. Venereol.* 1996;76:169-70.

Olszewska M, Kolacinska-Strasz Z, Sulej J, et al. Efficacy and safety of cyclophosphamide, azathioprine, and cyclosporine (ciclosporin) as adjuvant drugs in pemphigus vulgaris. *Am. J. Clin. Dermatol.* 2007; 8:85-92.

Oursler JR, Labib RS, Ariss-Abdo L, Burke T, O'Keefe EJ, Anhalt GJ. Human autoantibodies against desmoplakins in paraneoplastic pemphigus. *J. Clin. Invest.* 1992; 89:1775-82.

Pandya AG, Sontheimer RD. Treatment of pemphigus vulgaris with pulse intravenous cyclophosphamide. *Arch. Dermatol.* 1992; 128:1626-30.

Pantanowitz L, Fruh K, Marconi S, Moses AV, Dezube BJ. Pathology of rituximab-induced Kaposi sarcoma flare. *BMC Clin. Pathol.* 2008 Jul 23; 8:7.

Parnicka Z, Svecova D, Javor J, Shawkatova I, Buc M. High susceptibility to pemphigus vulgaris due to HLA-DRB1*14:54 in the Slovak population. *Int. J. Immunogenet.* 2013; 40:471-5.

Patsatsi A, Sotirious E, Devliotou-Panagiotidou D, Sotiriadis D. Pemphigus vulgaris affecting 19 nails. *Clin. Exp. Dermatol.* 2009; 34:202-5.

Patsatsi A, Kyriakou A, Giannakou A, Pavlitou-Tsiontsi A, Lambropoulos A, Sotiriadis D. Clinical significance of anti-demoglein-1 and -3 circulating autoantibodies in pemphigus patients measured by area index and intensity score. *Acta Derm. Venereol.* 2014; 94:203-6.

Peterson JD, Chan LS. Effectiveness and side effects of anti-CD20 therapy for autoantibody-mediated blistering skin diseases: a comprehensive survey of 71 consecutive patients from the initial use to 2007. *Ther. Clin. Risk Manag.* 2009; 5:1-7.

Pigozzi B, Pesericco A, Shiesari L, Alaibac M. Pemphigus foliaceus evolving into pemphigus vulgaris: a probable example of 'intermolecular epitope spreading' confirmed by enzyme-linked immunosorbent assay study. *J. Eur. Acad. Dermatol. Venereol.* 2008; 22:242-4.

Rahbar Z, Daneshpazhooh M, Mirshams-Shahshahani M, et al. Pemphigus disease activity measurements: pemphigus disease area index, autoimmune bullous skin disorder intensity score, and pemphigus vulgaris activity score. *JAMA Dermatol.* 2014; 150:266-72.

Rallis E, Stavropoulos P, Christofidou E, Rigopoulos D, Koumantaki-Mathioudaki E. Pemphigus vulgaris with plaque-type psoriasis successfully treated with cyclosporine monotherapy. *Am. J. Clin. Dermatol.* 2011; 12:283-4.

Robinson ND, Hashimoto T, Amagai M, Chan LS. The new pemphigus variants. *J. Am. Acad. Dermatol.* 1999; 40:649-71.

Rock B, Labib RS, Diaz LA. Monovalent Fab' immunoglobulin fragments from endemic pemphigus foliaceus autoantibodies reproduce the human disease in neonatal Balb/c mice. *J. Clin. Invest.* 1990; 85:296-9.

Rose NR and Bona C. Defining criteria for autoimmune diseases (Witebsky's postulates revisited. *Immunol. Today* 1993; 14:426-30.

Saha M, Harman K, Mortimer NJ, et al. Pemphigus vulgaris in White Europeans is linked with HLA Class II allele HLA DRB1*1454 but not DRB1*1401. *J. Invest. Dermatol.* 2010; 130:311-4.

Saha M, Bhogal B, Black MM, Cooper D, Vaughan RW, Groves RW. Prognostic factors in pemphigus vulgaris and pemphigus foliaceus. *Br. J. Dermatol.* 2014; 170:116-22.

Salato VK, Hacker-Foegen MK, Lazarova Z, Fairley JA, Lin MS. Role of intramolecular epitope spreading in pemphigus vulgaris. *Clin. Immunol.* 2005; 116:54-64.

Sarig O, Bercovici S, Zoller L, et al. population-specific association between a polymorphic variant in ST18, encoding a pro-apoptotic molecule, and pemphigus vulgaris. *J. Invest. Dermatol.* 2012; 132:1798-805.

Saruta H, Ishii N, Teye K, et al. Two cases of pemphigus vegetans with IgG anti-desmocollin 3 antibodies. *JAMA Dermatol.* 2013; 149:1209-13.

Schmidt E, Gutberlet J, Siegmund D, Berg D, Wajant H, Waschke J. Apoptosis is not required for acantholysis in pemphigus vulgaris. *Am. J. Physiol. Cell Physiol.* 2009; 296:C162-72.

Shams S, Amirzargar AA, Yousefi M, et al. HLA class II (DRB, DQA1, DQB1) allele and haplotype frequencies in the patients with pemphigus vulgaris. *J. Clin. Immunol.* 2009; 29:175-9.

Sharma VK, Khandpur S. Evaluation of cyclophosphamide pulse therapy as an adjuvant to oral corticosteroid in the management of pemphigus vulgaris. *Clin. Exp. Dermatol.* 2013; 38:659-64.

Sheehan DJ, Lesher JL Jr. Deep venous thrombosis after high-dose intravenous immunoglobulin in the treatment of pemphigus vulgaris. *Cutis* 2004; 73:403-6.

Shetty S, Ahmed AR. Preliminary analysis of mortality associated with rituximab use in autoimmune diseases. *Autoimmunity* 2013; 46:487-96.

Shivaswamy KN, Thappa DM. Extensive keloids following cyclosporine therapy in a pemphigus vulgaris patient. *J. Eur. Acad. Dermatol. Venereol.* 2007; 21:111-2.

Sinha AA, Hoffman MB, Janicke EC. Pemphigus vulgaris: approach to treatment. *Eur. J. Dermatol.* 2015; 25:103-13.

Spindler V, Drenckhahn D, Zillikens D, Waschke J. Pemphigus IgG causes skin splitting in the presence of both desmoglein 1 and desmoglein 3. *Am. J. Pathol.* 2007; 171:906-916.

Spindler V, Vielmuth F, Schmidt E, Rubenstein DS, Waschke J. Protective endogenous cyclic adenosine 5'-monophosphate signaling triggered by pemphigus autoantibodies. *J. Immunol.* 2010; 185:6831-8.

Stanley JR, Yaar M, Hawley-Nelson P, Katz SI. Pemphigus autoantibodies identify a cell surface glycoprotein synthesized by human and mouse keratinocytes. *J. Clin. Invest.* 1982; 70:281-8.

Stieger M, Pelivani N, Ramelet AA, Beltraminelli H, Borradori L. Penile erosions as first manifestation of pemphigus vulgaris: a misleading presentation. *Acta Derm. Venereol.* 2013; 93:248-9.

Tajima M, Mitsuhashi Y, Irisawa R, Amagai M, Hashimoto T, Tsuboi R. IgA pemphigus reacting exclusively to desmoglein 3. *Eur. J. Dermatol.* 2010; 20:626-9.

Takahashi H, Kuwana M, Amagai M. A single helper T cell clone is sufficient to commit polyclonal naïve B cells to produce pathogenic IgG in experimental pemphigus vulgaris. *J. Immunol.* 2009; 182:1740-5.

Takahashi H, Kouno M, Nagao K, et al. Desmoglein 3-specific CD4+ T cells induce pemphigus vulgaris and interface dermatitis in mice. *J. Clin. Invest.* 2011; 121:3677-88.

Tichy M, Urbanek J, Sternbersky J, Ditrichova D, Hercogova J. Life-threatening course of pemphigus vulgaris complicated by sepsis caused by azathioprine-induced bone marrow suppression, successfully managed with combination therapy. *Dermatol. Ther.* 2014; 27:183-6.

Tran KD, Wolverton JE, Soter NA. Methotrexate in the treatment of pemphigus vulgaris: experience in 23 patients. *Br. J. Dermatol.* 2013; 169:916-21.

Tunca M, Musabak U, Saqkan RI, Koc E, Akar A. Association of human leukocyte antigen class II alleles with pemphigus vulgaris in a Turkish population. *J. Dermatol.* 2010; 37:246-50.

Uludag HA, Uysal Y, Kucukevcilioglu M, Ceylan OM, Onguru O, Arca E. An uncommon ocular manifestation of pemphigus vulgaris: conjunctival mass. *Ocul. Immunol. Inflamm.* 2013; 21:400-2.

Uzun S, Durdu M. The specificity and sensitivity of Nikolskiy sign in the diagnosis of pemphigus. *J. Am. Acad. Dermatol.* 2006; 54:411-5.

Vasiliou A, Nikolopoulos TP, Manolopoulos L, Yiotakis J. Laryngeal pemphigus without skin manifestations and review of the literature. *Eur. Arch. Otorhinolaryngol.* 2007; 264:509-12.

Veraitch O, Ohyama M, Yamagami J, Amagai M. Alopecia as a rare but distinct manifestation of pemphigus vulgaris. *J. Eur. Acad. Dermatol. Venereol.* 2013; 27:86-91.

Vinay K, Kanwar AJ, Mittal A, Dogra S, Minz RW, Hashimoto T. Intralesional rituximab in the treatment of refractory oral pemphigus vulgaris. *JAMA Dermatol.* 2014; Dec. 23. Doi:10.1001/jamadermatol. 2014.3674.

Wang J, Kwon J, Ding X, Fairley JA, Woodley DT, Chan LS. Nonsecretory IgA1 autoantibodies targeting desmosomal component desmoglein 3 in intraepidermal neutrophilic IgA dermatosis. *Am. J. Pathol.* 1997; 150:1901-7.

Weber R, Monteiro F, Preuhs-Filho G, Rodrigues H, Kalil J, Miziara ID. HLA-DRB1*04:02, DRB1*08:04 and DRB1*14 alleles associated to pemphigus vulgaris in southeastern Brazilian population. *Tissue Antigens* 2011; 78:92-3.

Weinder GJ. Rituximab: mechanism of action. *Semin. Hematol.* 2010; 47:115-23.

Weiss D, Risti R, Griss J, et al. Autoantibody levels and clinical disease severity in patients with pemphigus: Comparison of aggregated anti-desmoglein ELISA values and indirect immunofluorescence titres. *Act. Derm. Venereol.* 2015; 95:559-64.

Wilgram GF, Caulfield JB, Lever WF. An electron microscopic study of acantholysis in pemphigus vulgaris. *J. Invest. Dermatol.* 1961; 36:373-82.

Wilson JP, Koren JF, Daniel RC 3rd, Chapman SW. Cefadroxil-induced ampicillin-exacerbated pemphigus vulgaris: case report and review of the literature. *Drug Intell Clin. Pharm.* 1986; 20:219-23.

Yamagami J, Payne AS, Kacir S, Ishii K, Siegel DL, Stanley JR. Homologous regions of autoantibody heavy chain complementarity-determining region 3 (H-CDR3) in patients with pemphigus cause pathogenicity. *J. Clin. Invest.* 2010; 120:4111-7.

Yan L, Wang JM, Zheng K. Association between HLA-DRB1 polymorphisms and pemphigus vulgaris: a meta-analysis. *Br. J. Dermatol.* 2012; 167:768-77.

Yoshimura K, Ishii N, Hamada T, et al. Clinical and immunological profiles in 17 Japanese patients with drug-induced pemphigus studied at Kurume University. *Br. J. Dermatol.* 2014; 171:544-53.

Zakka LR, Shetty SS, Ahmed AR. Rituximab in the treatment of pemphigus vulgaris. *Dermatol Ther (Heidelb)* 2012; 2:17.

Zhao M, Huang W, Zhang Q, et al. Aberrant epigenetic modifications in peripheral blood mononuclear cells from patients with pemphigus vulgaris. *Br. J. Dermatol.* 2012; 167:523-31.

Zhu X, Pan J, Yu Z, Wang Y, Cai L, Zheng S. Epidemiology of pemphigus vulgaris in the Northeast China: a 10-year retrospective study. *J. Dermatol.* 2014; 41:70-5.

Zillikens D, Rose PA, Balding SD, et al. Tight clustering of extracellular BP180 epitopes recognized by bullous pemphigoid autoantibodies. *J. Invest. Dermatol.* 1997; 109:573-9.

Zone JJ, Taylor TB, Kadunce DP, Meyer LJ. Identification of the cutaneous basement membrane zone antigen and isolation of antibody in linear immunoglobulin A bullous dermatosis. *J. Clin. Invest.* 1990; 85:812-20.

Index

A

B

C

D

M

N

O

P

R

S

T

U

V

W

Y